Feminist Action Research in Mental Health

Michele Jarldorn
Nicole Moulding • Kate Deuter
Editors

Feminist Action Research in Mental Health

A Practical Guide

palgrave
macmillan

Editors
Michele Jarldorn
University of South Australia
Magill, SA, Australia

Nicole Moulding
University of South Australia
Magill, SA, Australia

Kate Deuter
University of South Australia
Magill, SA, Australia

ISBN 978-3-032-04405-1 ISBN 978-3-032-04406-8 (eBook)
https://doi.org/10.1007/978-3-032-04406-8

This Palgrave Macmillan imprint is published by the registered company Springer Nature Switzerland AG.
The registered company address is: Gewerbestrasse 11, 6330 Cham, Switzerland

Preface

Gendered violence and other forms of gender inequality play a significant role in the mental health problems faced by young women; however, evidence suggests that many young women do not seek help. Whilst new and emerging digital and online mental health resources hold great promise as an adjunct to traditional face-to-face mental health support, they are predominantly designed for mixed gender audiences and do not connect young women's mental health with their gendered lived experiences.

In academic contexts, there has been a recent surge in feminist co-design initiatives where the focus is on collaborative and community-led research approaches and methods. However, scholars argue that the *translation* of feminist theory into research practices has been slow to transpire. What is missing so far in the published literature are specific examples of *both* the theory and the practice of co-designing feminist-informed online mental health applications with young women. This book presents the processes and results of a two-year study exploring young women's mental health using feminist participatory action research conducted in Australia; however, the approach we took, the results and the outcomes have broader implications for feminist responses to women's mental health challenges.

This book seeks to respond to this critical gap in theoretical and practical knowledge as it takes the reader through the development of an innovative, feminist-informed mental health peer support website co-designed with, and for, young women. Our research is grounded in feminist activism and is shaped by our commitment to a feminist ethics of care as it takes young women's gendered experiences of mental distress seriously. Our inclusive and participatory approach includes a dedicated chapter that invites the young women who participated in our study to share their personal experiences of collaborating in a co-designed research study.

We wrote this book with first-time and early-career researchers across the social sciences in mind, but also for those interested in co-design and those working in website design and have tried to make the work relevant to people outside academia. This means that we have used accessible language, without simplifying the content or the arguments made. If you are contemplating conducting a research project with co-design aspects using a feminist framework, but don't know where to start, we think this book will become a useful guide.

Magill, SA, Australia Michele Jarldorn
Magill, SA, Australia Nicole Moulding
Magill, SA, Australia Kate Deuter

Acknowledgements

We wish to acknowledge the Aboriginal and Torres Strait Islander peoples across Australia as the Custodians of this Country for the last 60,000 years. As residents of South Australia, we acknowledge the Kaurna, Boandik and Barngarla First Nations Peoples and their Elders past and present, who are the Traditional Owners of the lands that are now home to the University of South Australia's campuses in Adelaide, Mount Gambier and Whyalla. We also acknowledge the other First Nations peoples and lands across Australia, their Elders, ancestors, culture and heritage. Sovereignty has never been ceded.

There are many people to thank for helping us turn the idea for this book into a reality. Most important to recognise are the young women across Australia who responded to our survey and volunteered to participate in our online focus groups. We would especially like to thank the five young women who worked with us across the project to design and create the peer2me website.

This book, and this research project would not have been possible without the financial support of The Breakthrough Mental Health Research Foundation. We'd especially like to thank the Breakthrough Foundation's CEO John Mannion and media officer Tom Bell, both of whom supported us and the project across two years. Thank you to the team at Palgrave for supporting us in taking this book from an idea to the finished product. We are grateful for the ongoing support of the University of South Australia and especially our colleagues across our unique grouping of disciplines in the Justice and Society Academic Unit.

Contents

Notes on Contributors

Jane Andrew is the director of CoolBus Creative, where she collaborates with like-minded businesses to foster innovation and collaboration across professional disciplines. She describes herself as a 'Pracademic' who, over her career, has gained valuable insights into the diverse social, political, policy, professional and operational environments which shape people's lives.

Rosie Dale is a young white ciswoman with lived experience of severe mental illness and recovery. She is living with depression and anxiety, and has experienced an eating disorder, self-harm and suicidality. Her journey with mental illness has inspired her career choices and influenced her passions. Rosie writes from her experiences as a peer worker for metropolitan youth mental health NGOs and as a peer researcher who assisted in evaluating state and commonwealth suicide prevention initiatives.

Kate Deuter is a research associate at the University of South Australia. Her research is underpinned by co-design principles and aims to collaboratively develop solutions to social issues, including the impact of gendered violence, post-parental care planning needs of adults with intellectual disabilities in rural areas and mental health help-seeking of people from farming communities.

Abbey Hood lives and works on Peramangk Country in the Adelaide Hills. She is committed to trauma-informed, anti-oppressive and rights-based practice, with a particular interest in how gender, power and systems shape people's experiences. Drawing on experience across frontline and macro-level roles, she brings a strong feminist lens to both practice and policy. She is passionate about creating accessible tools that empower children, families and practitioners alike.

Michele Jarldorn lives and works on the unceded lands of the Kaurna people of the Adelaide Plains in South Australia. Her research uses an intersectional lens to connect structural violence with social problems. She is committed to privileging the perspectives and voices of research participants through the use of participatory, inclusive research methods with a social justice focus. Recently, her work has centred on co-designing tech for social good.

Jasmine Lloyd is a young woman living in Melbourne. She cares deeply about mental health, shaped by her own experiences and challenges. Jasmine was born extremely preterm and draws on this lived experience as a volunteer for a local not-for-profit and is part of a lived experience advisory group for clinical research in prematurity. Jasmine wishes that those struggling with mental health could access help that she and her loved ones couldn't find and wants to help improve outcomes for others navigating everyday mental health battles. She's found meaning in giving back through co-creating the Peer2me website.

Nicole Moulding is Professor of Social Work at the University of South Australia and Director of the Social Relationships and Communities Research Group. A researcher and educator with interests in gendered violence, mental health and social work, she has published three books and over 50 journal articles and book chapters across these fields.

Kirstie Wyatt has enjoyed over 30 years as a freelance graphic and web designer/developer and educator. She is based in Adelaide but works with clients globally. As director of Wyatt Creative, Kirstie delivers design services, including branding and logo design, magazine and other print collateral, event management, photo editing, web design and development, and email and digital marketing. Kirstie believes that excellent communication is one of the most important parts of the creative process, and her strength in this area has led to many regular clients who come back to her time and time again.

Kizzy Yang lives on the unceded lands of the Gadigal people in New South Wales. She is a speech pathologist, mental health advocate and lived experience advisor. Her work centres on the intersection of communication, trauma and mental health, with a focus on trauma-informed practice. Drawing on her lived experience, Kizzy supports more inclusive, relational and collaborative approaches in research and care. She is passionate about amplifying the voices of people with lived experience and advocating for systems that honour safety, dignity and connection.

CHAPTER 1

What Is Co-Design and Why Use It for Mental Health Research?

Michele Jarldorn, Nicole Moulding, and Kate Deuter

Abstract This chapter provides an introductory overview of the rationale for our co-designed action research project, which explores the scope of mental health peer support among young women. We begin by demonstrating the strong correlation between gender inequality, including experiences of gendered violence, and the mental health struggles faced by young women in Australia and other countries. We introduce the mixed-methods and participatory, action-oriented research design we employed, and make an argument for the benefits of using a co-design approach with young women. The language and tone used throughout the chapter purposefully seeks to demystify co-design research methods, especially for post-graduate and early-career researchers in social work and other social science disciplines.

Keywords Young women • Mental health • Gendered violence • Co-design

M. Jarldorn (✉) · N. Moulding · K. Deuter
University of South Australia, Magill, SA, Australia
e-mail: Michele.jarldorn@unisa.edu.au;
Nicole.Moulding@unisa.edu.au; Kate.Deuter@unisa.edu.au

M. Jarldorn et al. (eds.), *Feminist Action Research in Mental Health*, https://doi.org/10.1007/978-3-032-04406-8_1

Why Young Women and Mental Health?

As educators in disciplines such as social work that have large student cohorts of young women from diverse social backgrounds, we have observed over many years growing levels of psychological distress in our university classrooms. We wanted to understand what we were seeing and commenced by consulting the findings of the Household, Income and Labour Dynamics in Australia (HILDA) study findings, one of the largest longitudinal health research projects in the world (Wilkins et al., 2023). The HILDA study is an ongoing research project that follows the lives of over 17,000 Australians each year using a longitudinal study that draws on a large representative sample; as such, it is a highly credible, valid and reliable data source. The findings from the HILDA study point to a steady increase in the proportion of young people experiencing psychological distress. The report notes that since 2011, and particularly for young people aged between 15 and 24, the rate of disclosing psychological distress has more than doubled from under 20% to over 40%, while for the group aged between 25 and 34, at least a third of the group reported experiencing distress (Wilkins et al., 2023). However, the proportion of young Australian women reporting distress was far higher than for young men. While psychological distress does not necessarily refer to the diagnosis of a mental health condition, data from the Australian Bureau of Statistics' National Study of Mental Health and Wellbeing (ABS, 2020-2022) throws further light, reporting that, in 2021–2022, almost half of young women aged 16–24 years experienced anxiety, depression or substance misuse compared to one third of young men. This is a staggeringly high figure, yet much of the media reportage on the topic failed at the time to point out this gender disparity, as if it was somehow unremarkable, or perhaps expected, and therefore not worth mentioning. These disproportionate increases in psychological distress and mental health diagnoses among young women are not limited to Australia, either, with international studies showing much higher rates among young women compared to young men (Campbell et al., 2021; Dijkstra et al., 2024; Gagnè et al., 2022; Johansen et al., 2021; Stapley et al., 2025; Tseris, 2023).

We need to state from the outset that focusing on young women's mental health does not deny that young men also face problems. The point is that, as yet, there has been little attention to the question of *why* young women have suffered such disproportionately higher rates in recent years. This difference has often been flicked off as a case of young women being more open about their struggles than young men, but this claim does not stack up when the data sources are anonymised longitudinal population survey samples. Such a claim also assumes that young women are entirely comfortable admitting to mental health struggles, and this is not necessarily the case, either. Women struggling with poor mental health often face particularly negative reactions that cast them as hysterical and attention-seeking (Moulding, 2016), a major deterrent to any admission of difficulty. We will show that an epistemology of ignorance operates in relation to the crisis in young women's mental health, just as it does in many other areas of women's health (See Tuana, 1996). Perhaps most importantly of all, though, focusing on young women should not be understood as taking something away from young men. Many researchers concentrate on researching men's mental health, just as they should and including ourselves, exploring the ways male distress often (but not always) manifests in externalising behaviours such as drug and alcohol abuse, violence against other males and violence against women, including sexual violence, in turn increasing psychological distress among young women (Moulding et al., 2021). It is important to underscore, though, that while male distress is sometimes implicated in the perpetration of gendered violence, most perpetrators do not have mental health problems or histories as victims of violence (Maidment et al., 2024); male violence against women is perpetrated by a wide cross section of men and is enabled by intertwined structural and cultural unequal gender power relations (Franzway et al., 2019). Nonetheless, as contemporary feminists, we understand that men's experiences of the world, including of mental health and wellbeing, are also gendered (see Moulding, 2017). However, our purpose in writing this book does not include a dual focus on men's mental health or interrogation of their lived experiences in some misguided quest for 'gender equity' or 'even-handedness'. Interestingly, we are never asked to justify why we have not included women in our research into the gendered problems facing men but, in what has been described as 'whataboutery', we are very often challenged when our focus is on women, a phenomenon also noted by other feminist scholars (e.g., see McCabe, 2024; Taylor, 2023). Such experiences reflect the ongoing backlash against feminism that continues to confront scholars and activists to this day.

We should clarify that our focus on young women does not assume cisgender heterosexuality. In naming women, we are referring to all those who identify as women irrespective of their gender identity histories or sexualities. We are also aware that there are many individuals in the community who once lived as women and now identify as non-binary. While perhaps no longer identifying as female per se, they are likely to experience high rates of many of the gendered precursors to poor mental health experienced by young women; our book is therefore inclusive of, and addressed to, these groups, too. We take an inclusive approach and are well-aware that poor mental health is experienced at the highest rates of all by gender and sexually diverse individuals.

As feminist researchers and practitioners with a focus on women's gendered experiences of the world, we value the solidarity that comes with women working collectively to claim their rights. We see feminist research as an impetus for action and social change. As argued by Caroline Sweetman (2013), "feminist solidarity and collective action are founded on beliefs about individuals in engaging with others to bring about radical, visionary change, standing and acting together" (p. 217). Sweetman suggests that these ideals should underpin feminist research, while Wickstrom and colleagues (2021) propose that "feminist solidarity is a way of being that is embedded in cultural traditions and movements that resist women's socio-economic inequalities and patriarchal power" (p. 857). For us, there is a sense of (self) empowerment in researching from this position as it enables us to centre compassion and care within a relationship-based approach to working with people as favoured by social workers. A feminist perspective also brings with it a concern with the specific ways in which women's experiences of poor mental health are specifically gendered. This necessitates an exploration of the different ways that gender inequalities are scaffolded and built upon in a male-dominated gender order that has particular implications for women's mental health and wellbeing. It also necessitates focusing on the pathways forward *with* young women that build upon their agency and significant strengths.

Applying a feminist, action-oriented framework to our project enabled us to draw attention to the fact that too many young women's lives are steeped in abuse, violence, inequality and social injustice that bring serious implications for their wellbeing. Obviously, we are fully aware that abuse and violence are not lived interpersonally by every single young woman on the planet, but young women as a group arguably experience a level of structural violence at the hands of 'gender blind' social, health and legal systems historically designed around masculine norms and imperatives that often fail to account for women's needs over the life course.

Structural violence refers to the inequities and injustices embedded in social structures and institutional practices. It is a form of 'invisible' violence and is often activated through policy, welfare and service provision. As Pool and Geissler (2005, p. 63) explain, the effects of structural violence are felt most deeply by "those who are underprivileged: namely women, the poor, those of colour". Because structural violence is largely invisible, it often leaves individuals to internalise blame for their circumstances. Structural violence based on gender alone does exist and has been well-documented, gender also intersects with class, race, age and other social inequalities and identities, and these run deeply through every corner of society. However, while women's lives are complex and unique, and diverse groups bring diverse experiences, the gendered nature of women's lives in a male-dominated gender order will always involve a level of shared experience and commonality that reaches across identity groups. For young women, in particular, "violence is embedded in social life in multiple and complex ways, reverberating through women's lives to reproduce disadvantage and subordination" (Kidd, 2016, p. 42). A notable example are the restrictions on reproductive rights and autonomy that have been faced by women historically and more recently, particularly in the United States. Even before the overturning of Roe v Wade in the US Supreme Court in 2022 (Beddoe & Clarke, 2023), women's autonomy and constitutional rights have been diminishing in the US. Alarmingly, attacks on women's bodily autonomy are increasing on a global scale, including here in Australia (Baird & Flowers, 2024). These include a range of reforms that have disproportionately impacted women, with younger women particularly affected. For example, changed welfare provisions for sole parents during the 2010s have positioned young mothers as socially irresponsible scroungers (Wolfinger, 2022) with no acknowledgement that gendered violence often underpins the decision to leave relationships and that negotiating legal systems post-separation can represent the continuation of violence at a structural level (Laing, 2017). Indeed, the family law system in Australia has been described as "ground zero for misogyny" (Brandt, 2023, p. 404).

While structural violence often lies at the heart of many of the mental health problems faced by young women, the experience of accessing mental health care can compound psychological distress further, rather than ameliorate it. The language inherent in some relationships between people experiencing mental distress and more traditional healthcare providers can be understood as a form of symbolic violence, based as it so often is on gendered historical ideas about mental illness and related social stigma. The diagnosis of common mental illnesses is more common in women and risks "spoiled identities", judgement, segregation, loneliness and isolation (Alex et al., 2013). While there has arguably been improvement over the past two decades, stigma remains a powerful social mechanism with a long history in the response to mental illness. As Rössler (2016) states:

> The stigma attached to mental illness is ubiquitous. There is no country, society or culture where people with mental illness have the same societal value as people without a mental illness. (p. 1251)

Other more symbolic forms of violence against women that have implications for their mental health and wellbeing include the proliferation of narrow gender roles and expectations through advertising, media reportage and film (see, e.g., Davis et al., 2022), including the promotion of narrow beauty ideals, female sexualisation and socially constructed ideals of the 'good woman'. Arguably, these symbolic practices affect young women most of all, evidenced in high rates of eating disorders and body image dissatisfaction in countries like Australia (Moulding, 2016). These are just some examples of the intertwined structural and symbolic violences perpetrated against young women, all of which conspire against good mental health.

In recognition of the importance of language to mental wellbeing, we take care throughout the book to be inclusive because, as McLaughlin (2009) reminds us, "the spoken word carries more weight than its dictionary meaning" (p. 1102). We are mindful that the language around mental distress, mental health and gendered violence is nuanced and evolving, and that currently preferred terms may become contested within a very short timeframe. Take, for example, the language used for gendered violence. Often women are described as 'leaving', or as having 'left', a violent relationship. This assumes that the exit was planned, and that the outcome is an end to the violence when, in reality, women generally *flee* violence, and this is often a time when the violence in fact escalates. Despite the shift to the empowering language of 'survivor' rather than 'victim', surviving gendered violence does not necessarily mean the end of women's struggles (Adams et al., 2021; Moulding et al., 2021). Another cogent example that goes to language in the contemporary context pertains to the proliferation of trauma discourses in the mental health field. While mental health practitioners increasingly use the term 'trauma' and claim a 'trauma-informed' approach to practice, most mental health intervention remains situated within a psycho-medical paradigm that fails to recognise or challenge the structural and socio-cultural aspects of gendered inequality shaping women's mental health experiences. Rather than create significant change, this shift to the language of trauma can inadvertently lead professionals, family, friends and acquaintances to play into the neoliberal imperative that responsibility and choice lies with individuals rather than systems (Ross, 2022).

Context of Our Study

The overarching aim of this project was to investigate the potential of gender-responsive mental health peer support for young women in the Australian context. We chose to focus on peer support because it has been increasingly shown to be an effective approach to improving mental wellbeing that is cost-effective, accessible and centres the voices of those with lived experience. Before embarking on the project, we undertook a review of existing mental health supports and resources available in Australia, which revealed a lack of gender-specific, feminist-informed options. The project we developed on the basis of this review involved two distinct phases of research. The first focused on learning from young women whether there was an appetite for peer-informed resources and peer-to-peer support. The second sought to work from a collaborative and participatory approach to co-design an online resource with young women. Our approach was fundamentally informed by the view that mental ill-health is socially constructed and steeped in gender and other intersecting social power relations. We paid attention to the diverse social contexts young women live in, understanding that there is no one universal 'truth' about mental health/We were acutely aware of social power inequalities of gender, class and race, but also the inequalities between young women participants and ourselves as university researchers.

Other contextual factors also play a role in the decisions we make about research methodologies. When we set out to undertake this research, we did so in the context of the COVID lockdowns in Australia. Not only did COVID exacerbate the already increasing numbers of people reporting poor mental health, but it also changed the research tools we could safely use. This context encouraged us to shift away from face-to-face interviews and in-person focus groups, and to rethink how we bring research participants and their ideas together in other ways. After reviewing the available literature and scoping out the already available online mental health apps at the time, we launched an online qualitative survey (see Moulding et al.,

2024) in 2021. Although young women were welcome to contribute anonymously, they were invited to leave their contact details at the end of the survey if they were interested in participating in online focus groups. We used ZOOM to facilitate these groups, finding that for notwithstanding the difficulties, and sometimes impersonal nature of using video-conferencing software, this approach did enable us to reach women across wide-ranging geographical locations. While our research team was based in South Australia, where COVID was mostly contained and residents were able to move around with reasonable freedom, our participants were located across Australia, with some based in Melbourne, the capital city of the neighbouring state of Victoria, which had the lengthiest lockdown and enforced the strictest border controls in the entire world (Miller, 2021). We found that using ZOOM enabled the research team and our participants connect on the same level and in flexible ways. As Wahl-Jorgensen (2021) reflects, this choice can make ZOOM interviews "feel more relaxed and comfortable than their face-to-face equivalents" (p. 375).

Choosing a Research Methodology

If you are contemplating undertaking a co-design project, we encourage you to think critically about research methods and methodologies. Co-design research uses qualitative research almost exclusively and is often enhanced by the use of creative, arts-based, participatory and action-oriented approaches. The choice of tools and methods should be pragmatic, based on the method most likely to generate meaningful participation while gaining a deeper understanding of lived experience knowledge and the ways that social structures and culture shape this experience. While qualitative studies are sometimes criticised for smaller samples, the strength of qualitative research methods is their focus on depth rather than generalisability. Hence, more participants does not necessarily mean that the study will provide better insights or be more impactful. The idea that you need enormous samples to reach 'data saturation' can be outweighed by "information power", which can be achieved when the appropriate aims, a targeted sample, the 'right' questions and the most appropriate analytic strategy are deployed (Malterud et al., 2016).

There are myriad qualitative research tools that can be used to support a co-design project. Some examples include semi-structured interviews (Ahluwalia-Cameron, 2022), memory work (Michell et al., 2017), auto-ethnography (McWade, 2020), duo-ethnography (Emery & Jarldorn,

2025), qualitative surveys (Terry & Braun, 2017) and visual methods using artefacts to generate discussion (Mannay, 2015). Likewise, the range of arts-based methods is wide and includes photovoice (Jarldorn, 2018), collage and clay work (Buchanan, 2016) and video-journalling (Lewis et al., 2023). Creative methods can be powerful in their capacity to centre the perspectives of participants and can support you in answering your research question and addressing your research aims (Kara, 2020).

Positivist methods are grounded in the belief that knowledge can be discovered through empirical observation and measurement. However, positivist approaches tend to overlook subjective experience and the social context of people's lives and often prioritise objectivity and detachment over ethical considerations about equitable participation. Traditional positivist methods can also (wrongfully) come from the stance that the researcher's values and position in society do not influence the research undertaken. Conversely, researchers informed by feminist theory recognise the importance of positioning themselves in the research (Jackson et al., 2024). Researchers can go much further than merely positioning themselves, though. Feminist and social work researchers can use their research as resistance and a form of activism (Brown & Strega, 2015). Social work in all of its modes can be understood as a political practice. This combination of research and seeking change is also described as academic activism or 'schola[r]ctivism' (Rahbari et al., 2024); often, the more traditional research methods fail to capture the complexities of the human experience in society. However, it must not be assumed that research incorporating an activist stance is not simultaneously rigorous and devoted to developing a nuanced understanding of social phenomena and new ways to address them.

It is for the above reasons that we were interested in deploying methods that are participatory and inclusive. Inclusive participatory approaches to research depend on a particular mindset or way of thinking about the world and the capacity to apply that to the doing of the research. To maximise the inclusivity of our research, we adopt an intersectional feminist framework. While intersectionality is a term widely used in the contemporary vernacular, it is important to understand its roots in the work of Black feminist scholars. Although widely attributed to the work of legal scholar, Kimberle Crenshaw (1991) and sociologist Patricia Hill Collins (2000), Angela Davis's earlier (1981) book, *Women, Race and Class* explored the inequalities *between* women through her critique of elitism and racism found within the feminist movement and helps readers understand how class shapes women's lives, especially within families, relationships and religion. Intersectionality enables us to recognise that individuals simultaneously occupy multiple social positions and how these *intersect* to shape experiences and identity. Intersectionality can be used as a lens to examine power dynamics within and across social categories and can highlight how social hierarchies are produced through intersecting systems of power, privilege and oppression. Intersectionality considers how historical, cultural and structural contexts all play a role in women's gendered experiences but should not fall into ignoring gender as a powerful driver of inequality in its own right.

Co-design, co-production and participatory action research are terms that are often used interchangeably to describe research that generates new knowledge and new resources, services or products. Approaches to co-design are underpinned by two key rationales, one technocratic, the other democratic (Martin, 2008), however, there is "no universally agreed definition of what co-production is" (Pettican et al., 2023, p. 203). Rather, it is best to focus efforts on identifying the *practices* and *processes* that create the conditions for collaborative co-production (Pettican et al., 2023). The continuum of approaches ranges from consultation end product testing, right through to more inclusive (Jarldorn, 2022) and radical approaches (Jarldorn & Emery, 2024). Each of these are useful, but it is imperative that researchers be realistic about where their methodology sits across this spectrum.

Who Are We?

As we discuss throughout this book, co-design challenges the 'typical' arm's length, 'objective' researcher position, so it is important for our readers to get a sense of who we are, as our positionality determines how we have interpreted the literature, our findings and shaped our writing.

Michele: I was a very mature aged student when I entered university to study social work after having been a client of social work services. Most of my adult life before university was spent in low-paying, but highly skilled, roles predominantly filled by women. Over the 30 years I had worked in the garment industry, I had made everything ranging from denim jeans, high fashion, wedding dresses, tailored suits and even motorcycle leathers. Sometimes that work was supplemented with welfare benefits, and working or not, I mostly lived hand to mouth.

Common to all of these roles was that we were working class with many of my colleagues coming from migrant and refugee communities. One of the benefits of being immersed in such a gendered profession was the comradery and support women give each other. I have now learned that as we sat and sewed together, we were doing our own feminist consciousness raising as we shared and learned how our gendered experiences crossed cultural and geographical borders. The women I worked with in each of these settings supported each other through times of struggle, but there were many good times where we celebrated success, birthdays and welcomed babies into the world. Despite the mundane work that damaged our skeletal systems, stiffened our muscles and strained our eyes, my most enduring memories from this 30-year career were how we laughed together, a lot.

Perhaps this helps explains why my research uses feminist qualitative research methods, tends to be based in community, and draws upon action-oriented, participatory and co-design methods. As a community organiser, volunteer and activist with a community group that supports formerly incarcerated women outside of my academic work, I can attest to the benefits of women working together to support each other. My research with formerly incarcerated women confirmed for me that when a community experiences research participation as rewarding and 'proof' that their knowledge and experience is valuable, often there is a visible shift in their understanding of the world and their perceptions of 'self'.

Nicole: I was half-way through my undergraduate social work degree when I discovered feminism. Up until that point, I had been vaguely aware that not all seemed to be fair and right in the world of gender relations, but I had not yet found the words for it. Like most if not all young women, I'd experienced sexual harassment in the workplace and on the street, came close to something worse a few times, and when growing up, I had seen the completely unequal division of domestic labour in most of the homes around me, including my own. But I had no words to describe what I was seeing. In the first two years of my social work degree, we learned all about Marx—everyone at uni was a neo-Marxist back then, about Weber, Freud, and other (almost always) male theorists. Something was missing. I did not yet realise that this something was half the population, the female half.

Then early into my third year of study, I was sitting on my couch one night in my inner city share house writing an essay on rape law and how sexual assault was dealt with in the courts. As I read on, I became increasingly horrified until the penny dropped, helped along by the wonderful feminist scholars who had written critical pieces about rape and sexual assault. With a shock, I realised that the legal system was inherently misogynist and sexist, and a woman's chances of getting a conviction for rape were vanishingly small. Even more shocking, the likelihood that she would instead be blamed loomed large. I recall the creeping anger that stole across me as the full realisation of systemic male dominance and sexist bias sunk in. That was the day I became a feminist.

Fortunately, in that same year of my degree, I was taught for the first time by feminist social work academics. At last, social work started to make real sense because that invisible half of the population and their experiences were suddenly being accounted for. Not only did my studies start to make sense, but so did my life. I went on a placement at a women's community centre, supervised by one of those wonderful feminist social work academics, and worked with fabulous women in all manner of programs including assertiveness training for women. We even got to exercise that assertiveness when a man tried to attend our training! The idea that we had rights was like new information, and the opportunity to choose what we wanted and say what we thought was thrilling.

I went on to work in feminist women's health centres, most of which no longer exist, and then turned to postgraduate study in gender studies, followed by a PhD focusing on the gendered nature of treatment and prevention programs for eating disorders. That took me into a Research Fellowship in gender and mental health, and that then led into an academic social work position. I am still researching in the areas of women's health and gendered violence with many excellent feminist colleagues, including Michele and Kate.

Kate: As a 'late bloomer' to further study, I commenced my first university degree at the age of 26. Although one of my program preferences was for Professional Writing and Communication (given an interest in journalism and a brief stint at a well-known Adelaide newspaper as a teenager) After a last-minute offer, I was accepted for my first preference—Bachelor of Applied Science, Human Movement (Sports Science).. Admittedly, I struggled terribly with the 'hard science' courses, and by the one-and-a-half-year mark, I was losing momentum. I was 'called into the office' for a meeting with the program director. It was make or break time. What I didn't know then was that I would finally 'find my niche' in the program.

In mid-2006, I returned to university as a part-time Research Assistant. I became interested in qualitative research, especially in mental health settings. This led to my doctoral study which explored the meanings that older people attribute to protective factors that give them reasons and experiences to live following a suicide attempt. I graduated with my PhD in 2018. A shift to teaching and research within the discipline of social work saw my lens dramatically turn from a specific health focus towards more vulnerable and marginalised populations (including children and young people). Whilst this shift represented another key opportunity to 'find my niche', my involvement in the present study was met with some challenges. I had never conducted research with young women and despite having tutored hundreds of young women in numerous social work courses, I still had some trepidation about this. Having already worked on another co-design study, I was aware of the critical importance of relationship-building throughout the life of a project. But given the gendered nature of this study, it felt different. In reflecting with the research team, we acknowledged the deep connections that were made, especially with the five young women who worked with us over a year in the co-design sessions, and the amount of 'emotional labour' we (all) contributed to foster and nurture those relationships. And I feel this was fundamental to the success of our research.

Overview of the Following Chapters

This book is divided into two parts. The first part explores the theoretical framework we crafted to shape our research methodology and uses this lens to review the literature relating to young women's gendered experiences of mental ill-health and to explore the use of peer-to-peer support. While participatory, co-design projects are organic and based on respectful and engaged relationships with the community, the strength of this approach is that it combines academic knowledge and the knowledge drawn from lived and living experience of the previous research and the people who have lived that. Accordingly, co-design facilitators must be 'across' the literature, not only to understand context and gaps in research, but to help them identify when explanations for people's experiences differ from those that are 'accepted' as universal and widely understood. Therefore, Chap. 2 provides a review of the literature explaining the context of women's mental health, which we unashamedly situate within an intersectional framework. Chapter 3 focuses on peer support for mental health. We then complete the first part with Chap. 4, which draws the connections between feminist thought and action-oriented feminist research.

The second half of the book focuses on the practicalities of doing the research. Chapter 5 provides an example of the findings from our project survey and online focus groups. In Chap. 6 we explore the creative methods we used to create a website wireframe in collaboration with our participants and explore the practicalities of co-designing a website with a website designer. In the final chapter, we are joined by some of the young women who participated across the project to hear how they experienced participation in the project. We hope that this book becomes a useful resource, especially for post-graduate students and early-career researchers to help them map out their own co-design process.

References

Adams, E. N., Clark, H. M., Galano, M. M., Stein, S. F., Grogan-Kaylor, A., & Graham-Bermann, S. (2021). Predictors of housing instability in women who have experienced intimate partner violence. *Journal of Interpersonal Violence, 36*(7–8), 3459–3481. https://doi.org/10.1177/0886260518777001

Ahluwalia-Cameron, A. (2022). Dissertation data collection during a global pandemic: Barking dogs, crying babies, and feminist social work. *Affilia, 37*(1), 20–25. https://doi.org/10.1177/08861099211048244

Alex, M., Whitty-Rogers, J., & Panagopoulos, W. (2013). The language of violence in mental health: Shifting the paradigm to the language of peace. *Advances in Nursing Science, 36*(3), 229–242. https://doi.org/10.1097/ans.0b013e31829edcf3

Australian Bureau of Statistics. (2020-2022). National study of mental health and wellbeing. *ABS*. https://www.abs.gov.au/statistics/health/mental-health/national-study-mental-health-and-wellbeing/latest-release

Baird, B., & Flowers, P. (2024, October 18). A South Australian Handmaid's Tale: Inside the room where a Trumpian abortion bill was narrowly defeated. *Crikey*. https://www.crikey.com.au/2024/10/18/south-australia-handmaids-tale-trumpian-abortion-bill/

Beddoe, L., & Clarke, E. V. (2023). A critical commentary: Abortion stigma standing in the way of reproductive justice. *Aotearoa New Zealand Social Work, 35*(4), 125–135.

Brandt, S. (2023). The myth of gender neutrality in family court: A clinician's perspective on determinations of "the best interest of the child". *International*

Journal of Applied Psychoanalytic Studies, 20(3), 403–434. https://doi.org/10.1002/aps.1838

Brown, L. A., & Strega, S. (2015). *Research as resistance: Revisiting critical, indigenous, and anti-oppressive approaches.* Canadian Scholars' Press.

Buchanan, F. (2016). Touching on emotions: Using clay work in a context of relational empowerment to investigate sensitive issues. In L. Bryant (Ed.), *Critical and creative research methodologies in social work* (pp. 189–206). Routledge. https://doi.org/10.4324/9781315574905

Campbell, O. L. K., Bann, D., & Patalay, P. (2021). The gender gap in adolescent mental health: A cross-national investigation of 566,829 adolescents across 73 countries. *SSM-Population Health, 13*, 100742. https://doi.org/10.1016/j.ssmph.2021.100742

Collins, P. (2000). Gender, black feminism and black political economy. *The Annals of the American Academy of Political and Social Science, 568*(1), 41–53. https://doi.org/10.1177/000271620056800105

Crenshaw, K. (1991). Mapping the margins: Intersectionality, identity politics and violence against women of colour. *Stanford Law Review, 43*(6), 1241–1299. https://doi.org/10.2307/1229039

Davis, A. Y. (1981). *Women, race and class.* Vintage Books.

Davis, T., Hogg, M. K., Marshall, D., Petersen, A., & Schneider, T. (2022). The knowing mother: Maternal knowledge and the reinforcement of the feminine consuming subject in magazine advertisements. *Journal of Consumer Culture, 22*(1), 40–60. https://doi.org/10.1177/1469540519889990

Dijkstra, L., Gülöksüz, S., Batalla, A., & van Os, J. (2024). Young adults, particularly young women, account for an increasingly large share of Dutch mental healthcare expenditure over the period between 2015 and 2021. *Epidemiology and Psychiatric Sciences, 33*, e48. https://doi.org/10.1017/s2045796024000404

Emery, S., & Jarldorn, M. (2025). Cards against academia: Playing the game of 'opportunities' through a feminist friendship lens. In A. Walker, H. Grimmett, & A. Black (Eds.), *Ludic inquiries into power and pedagogy in higher education* (pp. 220–234). Routledge.

Franzway, S., Moulding, N., Wendt, S., Zufferey, C., & Chung, D. (2019). *The sexual politics of gendered violence and women's citizenship.* Policy Press. https://doi.org/10.1332/policypress/9781447337782.001.0001

Gagnè, T., Schoon, I., McMunn, A., & Sacker, A. (2022). Mental distress among young adults in Great Britain: Long-term trends and early changes during the COVID-19 pandemic. *Social Psychiatry and Psychiatric Epidemiology, 57*(6), 1261–1272. https://doi.org/10.1007/s00127-021-02194-7

Jackson, K. F., Goodkind, S., Diaz, M., Karandikar, S., Beltrán, R., Kim, M. E., Zelnick, J. R., Gibson, M. F., Mountz, S., Miranda Samuels, G. E., & Harrell,

S. (2024). Positionality in critical feminist scholarship: Situating social locations and power within knowledge production. *Affilia, 39*(1), 5–11. https://doi.org/10.1177/08861099231219848

Jarldorn, M. (2018). *Photovoice handbook for social workers: Method, practicalities and possibilities for social change*. Springer.

Jarldorn, M. (2022). Centring participants' voices as inclusive research practice: Putting the voice into photovoice. In P. Liamputtong (Ed.), *Handbook of social inclusion: Research and practices in health and social sciences* (pp. 1351–1367). Springer. https://doi.org/10.1007/978-3-030-89594-5_72

Jarldorn, M., & Emery, S. (2024). Using radical co-design to create and develop a technology-based solution to improve post-release outcomes for formerly incarcerated women: LindaBot. *International Journal of Communication, 18*, 1246–1265.

Johansen, R., Espetvedt, M. N., Lyshol, H., Clench-Aas, J., & Myklestad, I. (2021). Mental distress among young adults–gender differences in the role of social support. *BMC Public Health, 21*, 1–14. https://doi.org/10.1186/s12889-021-12109-5

Kara, H. (2020). *Creative research methods: A practical guide*. Policy Press. https://doi.org/10.56687/9781447356769

Kidd, A. (2016). Networks of violence in the production of young women's trajectories and subjectivities. *Feminist Review, 112*(1), 41–59. https://doi.org/10.1057/fr.2015.48

Laing, L. (2017). Secondary victimization: Domestic violence survivors navigating the family law system. *Violence Against Women, 23*(11), 1314–1335. https://doi.org/10.1177/1077801216659942

Lewis, K., Hamilton, L. G., & Vincent, J. (2023). Exploring the experiences of autistic pupils through creative research methods: Reflections on a participatory approach. *Infant and Child Development, 33*(3), e2467. https://doi.org/10.1002/icd.2467

Maidment, K., Jenkins, K., Houlihan, M., & the Prevention United Youth Advisory Group (YAG). (2024). *The significance of gender-based violence as a key driver in young women's disproportionate experiences of mental ill-health*. Prevention United. https://anrows.intersearch.com.au/anrowsjspui/bitstream/1/22787/1/apo-nid328294.pdf

Malterud, K., Siersma, V. D., & Guassora, A. D. (2016). Sample size in qualitative interview studies: Guided by information power. *Qualitative Health Research, 26*(13), 1753–1760. https://doi.org/10.1177/1049732315617444

Mannay, D. (2015). *Visual, narrative and creative research methods: Application, reflection and ethics*. Routledge. https://doi.org/10.4324/9781315775760

Martin, G. (2008). Ordinary people only: Knowledge, representativeness, and the publics of public participation in healthcare. *Sociology of Health & Illness, 30*(1), 35–54. https://doi.org/10.1111/j.1467-9566.2007.01027.x

McCabe, L. (2024). How are feminist policy frames challenged and resisted, and with what effects? Exploring the Scottish domestic abuse policy case. *European Journal of Politics and Gender*, 1–30. https://doi.org/10.1332/25151088y2024d000000040

McLaughlin, H. (2009). What's in a name: 'Client', 'patient', 'customer', 'consumer', 'expert by experience', 'service user'—What's next? *The British Journal of Social Work, 39*(6), 1101–1117. https://doi.org/10.1093/bjsw/bcm155

McWade, B. (2020). Was it autoethnography? The classificatory, confessional and mad politics of lived experience in sociological research. *Social Theory & Health, 18*(2), 123–137. https://doi.org/10.1057/s41285-019-00090-4

Michell, D., Beddoe, L., Fraser, H., & Jarldorn, M. (2017). Solidarity and support: Feminist memory work focus groups with working-class women studying social science degrees in Australia. *International Journal of Qualitative Studies in Education, 30*(2), 175–189. https://doi.org/10.1080/09518398.2016.1242804

Miller, N. (2021, October 3). Proud or mad? Melbourne's marathon lockdown becomes the world's longest. *The Age*. https://www.theage.com.au/national/victoria/proud-or-mad-melbourne-s-marathon-lockdown-becomes-the-world-s-longest-20210930-p58w9w.html.

Moulding, N. (2016). *Gendered violence, abuse and mental health in everyday lives: Beyond trauma*. Routledge. https://doi.org/10.4324/9781315816630

Moulding, N. (2017). "Becoming a better man": Narrating masculinities after childhood emotional abuse. *Affilia, 33*(1), 39–55. https://doi.org/10.1177/0886109917729665

Moulding, N., Franzway, S., Wendt, S., Zufferey, C., & Chung, D. (2021). Rethinking women's mental health after intimate partner violence. *Violence Against Women, 27*(8), 1064–1090. https://doi.org/10.1177/1077801220921937

Moulding, N., Jarldorn, M., & Deuter, K. (2024). What do young women want? Using a qualitative survey to explore the potential of feminist-informed mental health peer support. *Qualitative Social Work, 23*(2), 224–241. https://doi.org/10.1177/14733250221131598

Pettican, A., Goodman, B., Bryant, W., Beresford, P., Freeman, P., Gladwell, V., Kilbride, C., & Speed, E. (2023). Doing together: Reflections on facilitating the co-production of participatory action research with marginalised populations. *Qualitative Research in Sport, Exercise and Health, 15*(2), 202–219. https://doi.org/10.1080/2159676x.2022.2146164

Pool, R., & Geissler, W. (2005). *Medical anthropology*. Open University Press.

Rahbari, L., Kramer, D., Deserno, M., Tse, T., & Matos, T. R. (2024). Activism and academia: An interdisciplinary dialogue on academic freedom and social engagement. *Journal of Higher Education Policy and Management*, 1–17. https://doi.org/10.1080/1360080x.2024.2390197

Ross, L. K. (2022). The survivor imperative: Sexual violence, victimhood, and neoliberalism. *Signs: Journal of Women in Culture and Society, 48*(1), 51–75. https://doi.org/10.1086/720413

Rössler, W. (2016). The stigma of mental disorders: A millennia-long history of social exclusion and prejudices. *EMBO Reports, 17*(9), 1250–1253. https://doi.org/10.15252/embr.201643041

Stapley, E., Labno, A., Ravaccia, G., Crease, M., Deighton, J., Brooks, H., Le, H., Atkinson-Ryan, C., & Edbrooke-Childs, J. (2025). My story and me: A narrative study of young women and girls' stories of their mental health and associated support. *BMC Psychiatry, 25*(1), 1–15. https://doi.org/10.1186/s12888-025-06923-z

Sweetman, C. (2013). Introduction, feminist solidarity and collective action. *Gender and Development, 21*(2), 217–229. https://doi.org/10.1080/13552074.2013.819176

Taylor, J. (2023, April 16). Stop asking me 'what about men?' What would Jess say? https://whatwouldjesssay.substack.com/p/stop-asking-me-what-about-men

Terry, G., & Braun, V. (2017). Short but often sweet: The surprising potential of qualitative survey methods. In V. Braun, V. Clarke, & D. Gray (Eds.), *Collecting qualitative data: A practical guide to textual, media and virtual techniques* (pp. 15–45). Cambridge University Press. https://doi.org/10.1017/9781107295094.003

Tseris, E. (2023). Placing women's mental health in context: The value of a feminist paradigm. *Australian Journal of General Practice, 52*(7), 449–453. https://doi.org/10.31128/ajgp-02-23-6715

Tuana, N. (1996). Revaluing science: Starting from the practices of women. In R. J. Nelson (Ed.), *Feminism, science, and the philosophy of science* (pp. 17–35). Springer Netherlands.

Wahl-Jorgensen, K. (2021). The affordances of interview research on Zoom: New intimacies and active listening. *Communication, Culture and Critique, 14*(2), 373–376. https://doi.org/10.1093/ccc/tcab015

Wickström, A., Lund, R. W. B., Meriläinen, S., Øyslebø Sørensen, S., Vachhani, S. J., & Pullen, A. (2021). Feminist solidarity: Practices, politics, and possibilities. *Gender, Work and Organization, 28*, 857–863. https://doi.org/10.1111/gwao.12689

Wilkins, R., Vera-Toscano, E., & Botha, F. (2023). *The household, income and labour dynamics in Australia survey: Selected findings from waves 1 to 21. The 18th annual statistical report of the HILDA survey*. Melbourne Institute: Applied Economic & Social Research, The University of Melbourne. https://melbourneinstitute.unimelb.edu.au/__data/assets/pdf_file/0008/4841909/HILDA_Statistical_Report_2023.pdf

Wolfinger, E. (2022). Australia's welfare discourse and news: Presenting single mothers. *Global Media Journal, 16*(1). https://www.hca.westernsydney.edu.au/gmjau/?p=1543

CHAPTER 2

Placing Young Women's Mental Health in Context

Nicole Moulding, Michele Jarldorn, and Kate Deuter

Abstract In this chapter, we provide a brief history of key approaches to mental illness in western countries, showing how feminists have pushed back on traditional psychiatric explanations and treatment models through research demonstrating the links between the psychological distress experienced by women and gender inequalities borne of the patriarchal sociocultural contexts in which they live. We specifically explore how gendered violence, as a key manifestation of gender inequality, shapes young women's mental health and how mainstream mental health services often fails to take into account the gendered nature of these experiences in their models of service delivery.

Keywords Young women • Mental health • History • Gendered violence and abuse

N. Moulding · M. Jarldorn (✉) · K. Deuter
University of South Australia, Magill, SA, Australia
e-mail: Nicole.Moulding@unisa.edu.au;
Michele.jarldorn@unisa.edu.au; Kate.Deuter@unisa.edu.au

M. Jarldorn et al. (eds.), *Feminist Action Research in Mental Health*, https://doi.org/10.1007/978-3-032-04406-8_2

Introduction

Traditionally, mental health research has been located within the psycho-medical paradigm, where the focus is on biological and psychological explanations with an emphasis on pharmaceutical and psychological interventions (see, e.g., Tseris et al., 2024). In this chapter, we provide a brief outline of the history of psycho-medical model approaches to mental illness, elaborating how feminists have pushed back on these traditional explanations and treatment models by and showing, instead, that much of the unequal burden of psychological distress carried by women, particularly young women, is linked to living in a male dominated gender order.

Women and Mental Illness: A Brief History

Historical treatments for mental illness prior to the late nineteenth century cast mental illness as a "disease of the soul" (Meadows et al., 2020). Many people believed that supernatural forces were at play when a person was mentally unwell, including the idea that evil or demonic spirits possessed the person (Meadows et al., 2020). Other explanations involved moralistic ideas about mental illness as a punishment from God for sinful behaviour, or the widely subscribed to notion that a curse had been placed upon the family (Coudert, 2014). Treatment in Britain before the nineteenth century often consisted of keeping the unwell person in a cage, like an animal, with only straw bedding to sleep on, or banishing them entirely from the community. Often, the focus of these practices was 'moral' correction and punishment (Meadows et al., 2020).

With the Enlightenment and the rise of science and rationality during the nineteenth century, mental illness, or 'madness', began to be understood as an organic, physical condition rather than the manifestation of a diseased soul or moral failing on the afflicted person's part. This understanding led to a shift from caging unwell people to the growth of mental asylums. In this period, those labelled 'mad' were seen to be irrational and, as such, were considered a societal threat; securing them in asylums away from the rest of the community therefore became the preferred approach to dealing with the mentally ill (Foucault, 1965, pp. 241–278). Often, these asylums were operated as profit-making ventures (see Scull, 2015, pp. 188–223) while, at the same time, increasingly taking on the characteristic features of a prison. Scull (2015) describes these 'madhouses' as

> infested with fleas and rats ...[.]... so cold and damp that many patients suffered from gangrene and tuberculosis; patients were also grossly abused by the attendants. Beating and whipping were widely employed, and female patients were frequently raped. (p. 191)

While the above quote points to gendered violence within the asylums themselves, there was less acknowledgement of its role in producing the distress that led women to incarceration in the first place. It is well-established now that, throughout history, women have experienced layers of highly gendered sexual, physical and emotional abuse and were often deemed 'mad' as a result (Scull, 2009; Ussher, 2011). However, in earlier periods, the role of gendered abuse in female distress was rarely acknowledged. Instead, femininity itself was understood to be closely linked with madness through the cultural associations of the feminine with irrationality, emotionality, immorality and lack of self-control, and masculinity with rationality, morality and self-control (Moulding, 2016). As such, then, many key psychiatric diagnoses in the past were saturated in gendered assumptions, most famously that of hysteria (Appignanesi, 2011; Scull, 2009).

Indeed, throughout the nineteenth century, madness itself was increasingly cast as a feminine preserve, described as the 'female malady' (Showalter, 1993) and represented through the idea of 'the mad woman in the attic' (Ussher, 1991). Women were particularly constrained in the Victorian era, widely viewed as physically and mentally frail, sickly, weak, dependent, non-sexual or overly sexual, too emotional or too outspoken. Hysteria was understood as an inherently feminine condition related in various ways to the pathologically predisposed female reproductive system rather than female oppression in Victorian society (Showalter, 1993).

Hysteria became a common medical diagnosis for women exhibiting symptoms of anxiety, shortness of breath, fainting, fluid retention, irritability, nervousness, loss of appetite for food or sex and, contradictorily or sexually 'forward' behaviour. Not uncommonly, women's hysteria was attributed to the idea that the female reproductive system was inherently pathological, sometimes drawing more specifically on the ancient notion of the 'wandering womb', that is, the belief that a woman's uterus could move out of place (Thompson, 2012). Women on the receiving end of such diagnoses were often sent to asylums. In this way, rather than casting them as bad and immoral, women's honour and reputation could be maintained by the diagnosis of a medical condition and committal to an asylum. For the families of the women deemed hysterical, the asylum offered a convenient and socially acceptable excuse for inappropriate, and potentially scandalous, behaviour (Scull, 2009).

A reliance on asylums continued through the first half of the twentieth century with mental illness increasingly understood through biological models alongside improvements in pharmaceutical treatments, but women nonetheless continued to be understood as naturally more prone to mental pathology. The 1950s saw, for the first time, a major pushback on the dominance of psychiatric discourses of mental illness. The anti-psychiatry movement during this period made the case that mental illness is a perfectly rational response to difficult and distressing social circumstances (Laing, 1959). R.D. Laing argued that defining complex social problems as mental illness diagnoses oversimplified problems that were often greater than the individual concerned, undermined the dignity of the person involved, and resulted in inappropriate care measures. While Laing did not specifically focus on women, his social theory of mental illness nonetheless provided some impetus for looking at the social contexts of their lives and the social expectations placed on them. However, approaches like Laing's have never made it into mainstream approaches to mental health, and the medical and pathologising approaches to mental ill-health largely remain.

The Diagnostic and Statistical Manual of Mental Disorders (DSM) has almost biblical status in psychiatry as the basis for diagnosis, prognosis and treatment for mental illness. The DSM is published by the American Psychiatric Association, and there have been five editions, the first in 1952 and the most recent fifth edition in 2013, known as the DSM-5. While every edition purports to be the definitive statement on mental illness, there are major changes from one to the next, with an ever-expanding list of conditions and, at the same time, the removal of other whole diagnostic categories, or major revisions of key symptoms and treatment protocols. As has been argued by Marecek and Gavey (2013), "As the DSM's authority has stretched into areas far beyond its competence, it has fallen victim to its success" (p. 4). Critiques of the DSM are wide-ranging and include financial conflicts due to panel member ties with the pharmaceutical industry (Cosgrove & Wheeler, 2013), its failure to adequately account for the social circumstances of individuals' lives, and its tendency to encroach on ever-wider phenomena so that experiences once considered normative become reconstructed as pathological.

Feminist Understandings of Women's Mental Health and Wellbeing

While the DSM has continued to extend its reach over the decades, so too, feminists have maintained the view that women's mental health in patriarchal societies cannot be properly understood without recourse to the gendered social context and inequalities of women's lives. As noted, female distress has long been interpreted through a lens of mental pathology that ignores the gendered social contexts in which the distress has arisen (Guerin, 2017). Feminists in the late twentieth century drew attention, instead, to the ways in which a patriarchal male-dominated gender order creates and exacerbates many of the problems women struggle with. As asserted by Meadows et al. (2020):

> Women's mental distress refers to the effect of the material, social and political constraints of their lives under the oppressive conditions of patriarchy. Their discontent is expressed through symptoms that have been interpreted as illness or disorder. (p. 7)

Rather than accident or an oversight, Ehrenreich and English (1978/2005) argue that the idea that female distress emanates almost entirely from the body and mind of the woman herself was "the ideology of a masculinist society dressed up as objective truth" (p. 5). Using a feminist intersectional lens to critique the individualist framework of the DSM, Marecek and Gavey (2013) argue that "distress and emotional wellbeing, as well as disadvantage and privilege, are distributed along intersecting axes of gender, racial/ethnic categorization, economic status, and sexuality" (p. 7). This idea is supported by the work of Jane Ussher (2011) and more recently, Mountain (2024) and Zirnsak et al. (2024). Ussher proposes that the higher incidence of diagnosing and treating women for 'madness' lies within a patriarchal framework underpinned by operations of power and control. Ussher does not discount the reality of women's experiences, though, arguing that their distress is not due to individual pathology, but is an understandable and reasonable response to gender inequality and oppression. Judith Herman's (1992) groundbreaking work in women's mental health in the 1980s and 1990s has been instrumental for its insight that gendered violence and abuse are often central to women's experiences of mental health problems and the need for a trauma-informed approach to treatment.

As we pointed out in the previous chapter, young women continue to carry a heavier burden of poor mental health across the globe than other groups in the population (Wilkins et al., 2019; World Health Organisation, 2020). Also as noted earlier, young women are two to three times more likely to report feeling mentally unwell than young men (AIHW, 2023); almost half report high levels of psychological distress (Mishra et al., 2014); one in five have been diagnosed with anxiety and depression (Wilkins et al., 2019); and 45% have reported self-harm (Holder & Fitzgerald, 2016). Young women in Australia aged 18–29 years also report the lowest levels of wellbeing of all groups (NAB, 2017), while those aged under 25 years continue to have the highest reported prevalence of mental health problems in the population (ABS, 2020–2022). While young women carry the heaviest burden of poor mental health, it is worth noting that the COVID pandemic further exacerbated poor mental health across the Australian community and that since that time there has been a general increase in rates of dispensing prescriptions for mental health related problems and an increase in calls to Lifeline, the Australian telephone crisis support service, (AIHW, 2023). During the last few years, a series of climate-related disasters and economic crises have also impacted on the capacity of mental health services across Australia. However, these population-wide events do not explain the disproportionate rises in poor mental health among young women.

While traditional psycho-medical models have long supposed that mental illness is largely caused by genetic propensity, despite a growing acknowledgement of multicausality (Cosgrove & Karter, 2018; Ferguson, 2017; Kökçinar, 2022; O'Connor et al., 2025), such explanations cannot account for recent increases in young women. Young women in particular have been long cast as 'naturally' prone to mental illness because of raging female hormones and a construction of female puberty as inherently unstable (Moulding, 2003, 2006). There is strong evidence, though, that the disproportionately poor mental health outcomes experienced by women across the life course, and the specific shape of these problems, are to a large extent a function of gender inequality (Andleeb et al., 2020; Moulding, 2016; Tseris, 2023), with widespread gendered violence the most serious and widespread contributor (Gibbs et al., 2018; Goncalves et al., 2022; Moulding et al., 2024; WHO, 2020). It is important to note that there has been an increase in sexual violence in Australia in recent years, with young women the most impacted group, as they are for all forms of gendered violence

(ABS, 2020–2022). Women who report both past and current male violence against them are highly likely to report psychological distress and related mental health diagnoses that have reverberating and compounding impacts on their access to work, income, housing and social participation (Franzway et al., 2019; Howard et al., 2010; Moulding et al., 2021). In the longer term, the survival strategies women rely on to keep themselves safe while living in abusive relationships may later serve to limit further their capacities to function socially, leading to persistent struggles with mental health and wellbeing that continue to reproduce the initial distress (Sinko et al., 2022).

While there is strong evidence that gender inequality and experiences of gendered violence increase the risk of mental health problems for women, particularly young women (White et al., 2024), this is not always appreciated in the general mental health literature or practice field (de Silva de Alwis, 2012; Maidment, et al., 2024; Moulding et al., 2021; Taylor, 2022; White et al., 2024; World Health Organisation, 2020). Moreover, despite the widely held belief that women are more willing than men to talk about, or seek help for, their mental health, evidence suggests that many do not access services (Scott et al., 2012) and, when they do, they often report that that services can be unhelpful, blaming them through responses that are rooted "in misogyny and sexism" (Taylor, 2021, p. 202). As Tseris (2023) points out, once women have had an unhelpful encounter when accessing mental health services or engaging with individual practitioners, this can lead them to resist engaging with professionals in the future. In combination with long waiting lists and greater appreciation of the benefits of lived experience and peer support, there has been growing interest from researchers and practitioners in the scope of peer led mental health support for women—including young women—as an innovative, cost effective and potentially more meaningful approach to engagement (Andleeb et al., 2020). We will discuss this later in the chapter, but first, we turn to examine the impact of gendered violence, both interpersonal and structural, on young women.

Gendered Violence, Abuse and Mental Health

Research evidence demonstrates a distinctly gendered pattern of individual mental health experiences after 13 years of age, with different types of problems affecting boys and girls, and girls generally reporting more mental health problems than boys (Barr et al., 2024; Winchester et al., 2022).

As noted earlier, explanatory models have traditionally focused on supposed biological differences between the sexes related to hormones, genetics or psychological functioning (Fullagar & O'Brien, 2012; Moulding, 2016; Ngun et al., 2011). Perhaps more commonly, much of the research into mental health among young people has failed to consider sex or gender at all, preferring a gender neutral approach that, at the same time, embraces a host of implicitly gendered assumptions about mental health and illness (Moulding, 2016). In contrast, research that takes a social view of health and wellbeing has explored how social circumstances impact individual mental health. This kind of research consistently finds that gender inequality and gendered experiences of stress, gendered violence and cultural norms contribute to the increased level of mental health problems experienced by women, particularly young women (Taylor, 2021; Landstedt et al., 2009). Arguably, then, acknowledging the social basis of the mental health challenges faced by young women is fundamental to providing effective care and the prevention of mental ill-health.

According to the World Health Organisation (2024), an estimated 30% of all women over the age of 15 who have been in a relationship have experienced gendered violence, while close to 40% of all murders of women were committed by a current or former partner. Gendered violence causes more death and disabilities, including psychological distress and diagnosable conditions, among women aged 15–44 years than cancer, malaria, traffic accidents and war combined (de Silva de Alwis, 2012; Moulding et al., 2023). Mental health conditions that have been specifically linked to just one form of gendered violence, intimate partner violence, include depression, anxiety and post-traumatic stress disorder (PTSD), as well as substance misuse and self-harm (Boyd et al., 2022; Romito et al., 2005; WHO, 2011). There is strong evidence that much of the heavier burden of common mental health problems carried by women across their lives is a direct consequence of intimate partner violence in particular (Buchanan & Humphreys, 2021; Taylor, 2021; Walby & Allen, 2004). Studies have also shown that women who report both past and current violence are almost six times more likely to report psychological distress than women who have not (Romito et al., 2005; Sinko et al., 2024), with coercive control known to have a particularly pernicious impact (Buchanan & Humphreys, 2021; Moulding et al., 2021; Scheffer Lindgren & Renck, 2008). Although recent debates have focused on defining what constitutes coercive control, usually as part of the process of criminalising perpetrator behaviour (Wiener, 2022), some have argued that "all violence is coercive and controlling" (Walby & Towers, 2018, p. 26).

More than one in two women who experience mental health problems are known to have experienced some form of violence or abuse (AVA & Agenda, 2017b; Scott & McManus, 2016). In a large national study (N = 658) conducted with women aged 18 years and over in Australia about the longer-term impact of intimate partner violence, over half (52%) reported that they had received a diagnosis of a mental illness, with over 40% diagnosed during intimate partner violence or after leaving; most were diagnosed with anxiety, depression or post-traumatic stress disorder (Moulding et al., 2021). This study also revealed that the diagnosis of common mental health problems in women who experience intimate partner violence is more than double the rate for women in the wider population (Moulding et al., 2021), providing a stark picture of the pervasiveness of the harms that intimate partner violence causes for women, most of whom had no history of mental health problems pre-violence. Importantly, gendered violence works to further exacerbate women's inequalities in relation to income, work, housing and social participation, ultimately undermining their capacities to function as equal citizens with rights to these social goods (Franzway et al., 2019). Despite the significant and long-term impact of gendered violence on women's mental health and wellbeing, this is rarely addressed in policy or service provision. For example, there is no mention of gendered violence, or any other form of gender inequality or discrimination, in the Australian government's National Mental Health Policy (Moulding et al., 2021).

Gender Inequality and Mental Health

In addition to gendered violence and abuse, a key risk factor affecting women's mental health is their socio-economic status, characterised by income inequality and reduced access to social and economic resources (AVA & Agenda, 2017a; Parra-Mujica et al., 2023), both of which are worsened by gendered violence (Franzway et al., 2019). Women also experience specific types of social marginalisation related to their gendered social roles, particularly the disproportionate burden of caring (Akkan, 2020; WHO, 2020); what has been described as the 'unremitting responsibility' for the care of others. Social isolation is another significant element in struggles with mental health and wellbeing, both as a contributor to the development of problems but also as a consequence of them (Bland et al., 2015). However, just like mental problems themselves, social isolation is also a highly gendered phenomenon (Mitchell & Smith, 2020) and is disproportionately experienced by women on the end of coercive control in intimate partner violence with often devastating impacts on wellbeing and suicidal ideation (Moulding et al., 2021). Social isolation is also significant after leaving intimate partner violence and can be associated with long-term difficulties around mental health and wellbeing (Franzway et al., 2018; Moulding et al., 2023).

Poverty itself is strongly associated with poor mental health, with women disproportionately represented among the poor (Smith & Mazure, 2021) and young women particularly affected (Agenda & AVA, 2019). The gender pay gap between women and men remains at over 11% (Workplace Gender Equality Agency, 2024), rising to around 30% for women who have children (Costa Dias et al., 2020), contributing to high rates of gender inequality and poverty among women. Women from diverse populations also face particular struggles around mental health, including minimisation of their experiences and silencing of their voices. Examples of diverse populations discussed in the Australian context include Aboriginal women who are victims of violence (McQuire, 2024), women from non-English speaking and culturally diverse communities and women who are refugees (Sullivan et al., 2020), formerly incarcerated women (Jarldorn, 2019), individuals who identify as women in the LGBTQIA+ community (Testa et al., 2017) and women who have a disability (Bend & Fielden, 2021). Importantly, in all of these sub-populations of women, young women carry particularly high risks.

Conversely, protective factors for the prevention of mental health problems parallel these risk indicators and include autonomy, access to material resources and feeling supported by others, such as family, friends, and health services (Maidment et al., 2024; WHO, 2020). Despite evidence about the numerous intersecting life stressors experienced by women accessing health and social care services, dominant service delivery models often fail to address the intersectional nature of the factors that contribute to poorer mental health for women (AVA & Agenda, 2017b. p. 5). However, while we acknowledge that women's experiences of mental health and wellbeing often involve intersecting identities and inequalities that complicate the picture, we are also arguing that gender, in its own right, brings particular challenges that are felt across all groups of women in a male-dominated gender order; this insight is key to an intersectional perspective because Crenshaw (1991) never meant that the *only* form of gender inequality is an intersectional one. At the same time, we acknowledge that gender inequality is *exacerbated* by intersectional inequalities.

Dominant Models of Mental Health Service Delivery

Within the illness-oriented psycho-medical model, consumers are often subject to a medical interpretation of their experiences that focuses on what is wrong with them rather than what is wrong with their situations (Mead & MacNeil, 2006). More specifically, as one of us has previously argued, "psycho-medical approaches assume and adopt a medicalized understanding of, and approach to, mental illness as real and definable 'disorders' that inhabit an individual body and are reflective of psychopathology in that body" (Moulding et al., 2021, p. 1066). Glover (2005) refers to this medicalised approach as relating to the person through the 'It' rather than the 'Me', an approach that encourages individuals to be passive recipients rather than active partners in their own care, and one that focuses on the permanency of disability rather than hoping for change. The limited scope of this focus risks reducing the capacity of individuals to manage their distress in empowered ways while, at the same time, undermining the ability of service providers and others to provide appropriate support.

As noted earlier, in addition to the risk of encountering pathologising, medicalised understandings of their problems, young women also continue to face persistent gender stereotypes that paint them as *inherently* emotionally unstable; this can mean that their difficulties are tolerated, discounted or dismissed in ways those of other groups are not (Moulding, 2016; Taylor, 2022), with young women with diverse and intersecting identities at greatest risk. For example, while hysteria no longer exists officially as a diagnostic category, some feminists argue that it is alive and well in the contemporary diagnosis and treatment of borderline personality disorder (Dorfman & Reynolds, 2023; Wirth-Cauchon, 2001; Shaw & Proctor, 2005). Understandings of what constitutes ideal mental health are also deeply gendered, exemplified in the famous 1970s study by Broverman and colleagues that demonstrated how the 'normal healthy adult' was envisioned by mental health practitioners as male, identifying behaviour considered 'unfeminine' and pathologised in women, while traditional feminine behaviours were cast as signs of mental illness (Broverman et al., 1970). As such, then, understandings of mental illness are very much gendered, and it is vital that the legacy of these historical discourses be understood in the contemporary context; they do not simply disappear within a generation or two. Because women, and young women in particular, are far more likely to be diagnosed with a common mental health problem than other groups, they are also far more likely to be on the receiving end of these pathologising notions of mental illness from treating professionals (Tseris, 2016, 2023). While a bio-psycho-social model has been dominant for many years now in recognition that mental health problems emerge from multidimensional causes, there has arguably been a focus on the biological and psychological at the expense of the social dimensions of mental health and wellbeing (Moulding, 2016). Further to this and as noted briefly earlier, psycho-medical approaches to mental health often take a 'gender-neutral' stance, blinding them to the gendered nature of experiences that are linked to poor mental health for young women, including gendered abuse (Moulding et al., 2021). For example, a cross-sectional survey of psychiatrists and psychiatric nurses in the UK found that mental health professionals experience difficulties in assessing and managing domestic violence, with 60% of professionals reporting a lack of knowledge about domestic violence support services (Nyame et al., 2013). Since this study was published, other researchers report similar results more than a decade later, pointing to no change (see, e.g., Vranda et al., 2023; Martinez-Garcia, et al., 2021; Tseris, 2024). Relatedly, though, while psycho-medical approaches are ostensibly gender-neutral, they are also deeply gendered in their assumptions about mental health and illness such that women are far more likely to receive a diagnosis and be prescribed psychotropic medication (Moulding, 2016; Ussher, 2011).

Conclusion

In this chapter, we have argued that effective mental health strategies cannot be gender-neutral when the risks faced are profoundly gendered and include everyday sexism and racism in concert with lower social status and life opportunities than those available to men. Moreover, supposedly gender-neutral approaches have been shown to be inherently gendered in their assumptions about mental health and illness. For too many young women, feelings of self-worth and personal competence, autonomy, adequate income and a sense of physical, sexual and psychological safety and security, all of which are essential to good mental health, have been systematically denied. Shifts are needed within traditional mental health services to gender-aware intersectional understandings of young women's mental health, wider challenges to systemic sexism and improvements to women's social, psychological and economic security and safety. Importantly, multi-level changes are required to improve wellbeing among young women, and these need to be approached as linked to each other. Hence, while peer support offers opportunities for young women to better understand how gendered violence and other forms of gender inequality impact on their mental wellbeing, new connections forged could also contribute to a new feminist activism on women's mental health. Such activism could challenge long-held assumptions that female distress, particularly that experienced by younger women, is mainly borne of hormonal imbalances and inherent feminine frailty, shifting attention instead to the intersecting gender inequalities and prejudices that underpin the higher rates of distress experienced by young women. Researchers can play an important role in advocating for critical feminist, social and intersectional approaches to mental health for young women, drawing attention to the need for governments, policy makers and practitioners to respond more appropriately and effectively.

References

Agenda, & AVA. (2019). *Breaking down the barriers: Findings of the national commission on domestic and sexual violence and multiple disadvantage*. https://weareagenda.org/wp-content/uploads/2019/02/Breakingdown-the-Barriers-full-report-FINAL.pdf

Akkan, B. (2020). An egalitarian politics of care: Young female carers and the intersectional inequalities of gender, class and age. *Feminist Theory, 21*(1), 47–64. https://doi.org/10.1177/1464700119850025

Andleeb, H., Parker, J., Mackay, T., Matthews, F., McWilliam, J., Haider, F., Iqbal, N., White, S., & Pinfold, V. (2020). *Evaluation of the women side by side project. Final report*. McPin Foundation and St George's University of London, UK.

Appignanesi, L. (2011). *Mad, bad and sad: A history of women and the mind doctors from 1800 to the present*. Hachette UK.

Australian Bureau of Statistics. (2020–2022). National study of mental health and wellbeing. *ABS*. https://www.abs.gov.au/statistics/health/mental-health/national-study-mental-health-and-wellbeing/latest-release

Australian Institute of Health and Welfare AIHW. (2023). *The health of Australia's females: Mental illness.* https://www.aihw.gov.au/reports/men-women/female-health/contents/how-healthy#mental_health

AVA, & Agenda. (2017a). *Mapping the Maze: Services for women experiencing multiple disadvantages in England and Wales.* https://www.mappingthemaze.org.uk/wp/wp-content/uploads/2017/02/Mapping-the-Mazefinal-report-for-publication.pdf

AVA, & Agenda. (2017b). *The core competencies of a gender sensitive service for women experiencing multiple disadvantage. A review of the literature.* AVA and Agenda.

Barr, M., Anderson, R., Morris, S., & Johnston-Ataata, K. (2024). Towards a gendered understanding of women's experiences of mental health and the mental health system. *Women's Health Issues Paper, 17*(2), 1–62.

Bend, G., & Fielden, S. (2021). I see you but you don't see me: The "two-way mirror effect" of gender and disability in employment. *Gender in Management, 36*(7), 821–838. https://doi.org/10.1108/GM-03-2019-0049

Bland, R., Renouf, N., & Tullgren, A. (2015). *Social work practice in mental health: An introduction* (2nd ed.). Allen & Unwin.

Boyd, J., Maher, L., Austin, T., Lavalley, J., Kerr, T., & McNeil, R. (2022). Mothers who use drugs: Closing the gaps in harm reduction response amidst the dual epidemics of overdose and violence in a Canadian urban setting. *American Journal of Public Health, 112*(S2), S191–S198. https://doi.org/10.2105/ajph.2022.306776

Broverman, I. K., Broverman, D. M., Clarkson, F. E., Rosenkrantz, P. S., & Vogel, S. R. (1970). Sex-role stereotypes and clinical judgments of mental health. *Journal of Consulting and Clinical Psychology, 34*(1), 1.

Buchanan, F., & Humphreys, C. (2021). Coercive control during pregnancy, birthing and postpartum: Women's experiences and perspectives on health practitioners' responses. *Journal of Family Violence, 36*(3), 325–335. https://doi.org/10.1007/s10896-020-00161-5

Cosgrove, L., & Karter, J. M. (2018). The poison in the cure: Neoliberalism and contemporary movements in mental health. *Theory & Psychology, 28*(5), 669–683.

Crenshaw, K. (1991). Mapping the margins: Intersectionality, identity politics and violence against women of colour.*Stanford Law Review, 43*(6), 1241–1299. https://doi.org/10.2307/1229039

Cosgrove, L., & Wheeler, E. E. (2013). Industry's colonization of psychiatry: Ethical and practical implications of financial conflicts of interest in the DSM-5. *Feminism & Psychology, 23*(1), 93–106. https://doi.org/10.1177/0959353512467972

Costa Dias, M., Joyce, R., & Parodi, F. (2020). The gender pay gap in the UK: Children and experience in work. *Oxford Review of Economic Policy, 36*(4), 855–881. https://doi.org/10.1093/oxrep/graa053

Coudert, A. P. (2014). Melancholy, madness, and demonic possession in the early modern west. In A. Classen (Ed.), *Mental health, spirituality, and religion in the middle ages and early modern age* (pp. 647–689). De Gruyter. https://doi.org/10.1515/9783110361643.647

Dorfman, N., & Reynolds, J. M. (2023). The new hysteria: Borderline personality disorder and epistemic injustice. *IJFAB: International Journal of Feminist Approaches to Bioethics, 16*(2), 162–181.

Ehrenreich, B., & English, D. (1978/2005). *For her own good: Two centuries of the 'experts' advice to women*. Random House.

Ferguson, I. (2017). *Politics of the mind: Marxism and mental distress*. Bookmarks Publications.

Foucault, M. (1965). *Madness and civilization: A history of insanity in the age of reason*. Vintage Books.

Franzway, S., Moulding, N., Wendt, S., Zufferey, C., & Chung, D. (2018). *The sexual politics of gendered violence and women's citizenship*. Policy Press. https://doi.org/10.1332/policypress/9781447337782.003.0001

Franzway, S., Moulding, N., Wendt, S., Zufferey, C., & Chung, D. (2019). *The sexual politics of gendered violenceand women's citizenship*. Policy Press. https://doi.org/10.1332/policypress/9781447337782.001.0001

Fullagar, S., & O'Brien, W. (2012). Immobility, battles and the journey to feeling alive: Women's metaphors of self-transformation through depression and recovery. *Qualitative Health Research, 22*(8), 1063–1072. https://doi.org/10.1177/1049732312443738

Gibbs, A., Dunkle, K., & Jewkes, R. (2018). Emotional and economic intimate partner violence as key drivers of depression and suicidal ideation: A cross-sectional study among young women in informal settlements in South Africa. *PloS one, 13*(4), e0194885–e0194885. https://doi.org/10.1371/journal.pone.0194885

Glover, H. (2005). Recovery based service delivery: Are we ready to transform the words into a paradigm shift? *Australian e-Journal for the Advancement of Mental Health, 4*(3), 179–182. https://doi.org/10.5172/jamh.4.3.179

Gonçalves Júnior, J., Maia, M. A. G., Moreira, J. L. de S., Dias, H. S., Félix, E. B., & Machado, S. S. F. (2022).Domestic violence against Latin American women and female mental health during the new coronavirus (SARSCoV-2) outbreak. *International Journal of Injury Control and Safety Promotion, 29*(2), 193–196. https://doi.org/10.1080/17457300.2021.1978101

Guerin, B. (2017). *How to rethink mental illness: The human contexts about the labels*. Routledge. https://doi.org/10.4324/9781315462615

Herman, J. (1992). *Trauma and recovery: The aftermath of violence—From domestic abuse to political terror*. Basic Books.

Holder, C., & Fitzgerald, D. (2016). *ALSWH data book for first survey of 1989–95 cohort. Australian Longitudinal Study on Women's Health*. https://alswh.org.au/wp-content/uploads/2020/03/2016_Technical-Report_39.pdf

Howard, L. M., Trevillion, K., & Agnew-Davies, R. (2010). Domestic violence and mental health. *International Review of Psychiatry, 22*(5), 525–534. https://doi.org/10.3109/09540261.2010.512282

Jarldorn, M. (2019). Radically rethinking social work in the criminal (in)justice system in Australia. *Affilia—Journal of Women and Social Work, 35*(3), 327–343. https://doi.org/10.1177/0886109919866160

Kökçinar, R. (2022). Climate change-related distress within the dominant mental health paradigm: Problems,pitfalls, and a possible way forward. *Psychotherapy and Counselling Journal of Australia, 10*(2). https://doi.org/10.59158/001c.71204

Laing, R. D. (1959). *The divided self*. Tavistock.

Landstedt, E., Asplund, K., & Gillander, G. K. (2009). Understanding adolescent mental health: The influence of social processes, doing gender and gendered power relations. *Sociology of Health & Illness, 31*(7), 962–978. https://doi.org/10.1111/j.1467-9566.2009.01170.x

Maidment, K., Jenkins, K., Houlihan, M., & the Prevention United Youth Advisory Group (YAG). (2024). *Policy brief: The significance of gender-based violence as a key driver in young women's disproportionate experiences of mental ill-health*. Prevention United. https://anrows.intersearch.com.au/anrows-jspui/bitstream/1/22787/1/apo-nid328294.pdf

Marecek, J., & Gavey, N. (2013). DSM-5 and beyond: A critical feminist engagement with psychodiagnosis. *Feminism & Psychology, 23*(1), 3–9. https://doi.org/10.1177/0959353512467962

Martínez-García, E., Montiel-Mesa, V., Esteban-Vilchez, B., Bracero-Alemany, B., Martín-Salvador, A., Gázquez-López, M., Pèrez-Morente, M. Á., & Alvarez-Serrano, M. A. (2021). Sexist myths emergency healthcare professionals and factors associated with the detection of intimate partner violence in women. *International Journal of Environmental Research and Public Health, 18*(11), 5568. https://doi.org/10.3390/ijerph18115568

McQuire, A. (2024). *Black witness: The power of indigenous media*. University of Queensland Press.

Mead, S., & MacNeil, C. (2006). Peer support: What makes it unique? *International Journal of Psychosocial Rehabilitation, 10*(2), 29–37.

Meadows, G., Farhall, J., Fossey, E., Happell, B., McDermott, F., & Rosenberg, S. (2020). *Mental health in Australia: Collaborative community practice* (4th ed.). Oxford University Press.

Mishra, G., Loxton, D., Anderson, A., Hockey, R., Powers, J., Brown, W., Dobson, A., Duffy, L., Graves, A., Harris, M., Harris, S., Lucke, J., McLaughlin, D., Mooney, R., Pachana, N., Pease, S., Tavener, M., Thomson, C., Tooth, L., Townsend, N., Tuckerman, R., & Byles, J. (2014). *Health and wellbeing of women aged 18 to 23 in 2013 and 1996: Findings from the Australian longitudinal study on women's health*. Women's Health Australia. https://alswh.org.au/post-outcomes/2014-major-report-health-and-wellbeing-of-women-aged-18-to-23-in-2013-and-1996-findings-from-the-australian-longitudinal-study-on-womens-health/

Mitchell, C., & Smith, A. (2020). The lives of girls and young women in the time of COVID-19. *Girlhood Studies, 13*(3), v–xi. https://doi.org/10.3167/ghs.2020.130301

Moulding, N. (2003). Constructing the self in mental health practice: Identity, individualism and the feminization of deficiency. *Feminist Review, 75*(1), 57–74.

Moulding, N. (2006). Disciplining the feminine: The reproduction of gender contradictions in the mental health care of women with eating disorders. *Social Science & Medicine, 62*(4), 793–804.

Moulding, N. T. (2016). *Gendered violence, abuse and mental health in everyday lives: Beyond trauma*. Routledge. https://doi.org/10.4324/9781315816630

Moulding, N., Franzway, S., Wendt, S., Zufferey, C., & Chung, D. (2021). Rethinking women's mental health after intimate partner violence. *Violence Against Women, 27*(8), 1064–1090. https://doi.org/10.1177/1077801220921937

Moulding, N., Chung, D., Zufferey, C., Franzway, S., & Wendt, S. (2023). Social participation after intimate partner violence: Investigating the impact on women's citizenship. *Violence Against Women, 29*(14), 2754–2774. https://doi.org/10.1177/10778012231196051

Moulding, N. Jarldorn, M., & Deuter, K. (2024). What do young women want? Using a qualitative survey to explorethe potential of feminist-informed mental health peer support. *Qualitative Social Work, 23*(2), 224–241. https://doi.org/10.1177/14733250221131598

Mountain, I. (2024). *Mental health and otherness: Intersections between gender, race, class and age*. Taylor & Francis.

NAB. (2017). *National Australia Bank wellbeing report Q1*. https://business.nab.com.au/wpcontent/uploads/2017/07/australian-wellbeing-survey-q12017.pdf

Ngun, T. C., Ghahramani, N., Sánchez, F. J., Bocklandt, S., & Vilain, E. (2011). The genetics of sex differences in brain and behavior. *Frontiers in Neuroendocrinology, 32*(2), 227–246. https://doi.org/10.1016/j.yfrne.2010.10.001

Nyame, S., Howard, L. M., Feder, G., & Trevillion, K. (2013). A survey of mental health professionals' knowledge, attitudes and preparedness to respond to domestic violence. *Journal of Mental Health, 22*(6), 536–543. https://doi.org/10.3109/09638237.2013.841871

O'Connor, C. A., Zufferey, C., & de Anstiss, H. (2025). Governing failed neoliberal subjects: Representations of women's mental health in Australian mental health policies. *Qualitative Social Work, 24*(1), 61–77. https://doi.org/10.1177/14733250231222020

Parra-Mujica, F., Johnson, E., Reed, H., Cookson, R., & Johnson, M. (2023). Understanding the relationship between income and mental health among 16-to 24-year-olds: Analysis of 10 waves (2009–2020) of understanding society to enable modelling of income interventions. *PLoS One, 18*(2), e0279845.

Romito, P., Molzan Turan, J., & De Marchi, M. (2005). The impact of current and past interpersonal violence on women's mental health. *Social Science & Medicine, 60*(8), 1717–1727. https://doi.org/10.1016/j.socscimed.2004.08.026

Scheffer Lindgren, M., & Renck, B. (2008). 'It is still so deep-seated, the fear': Psychological stress reactions as consequences of intimate partner violence. *Journal of Psychiatric and Mental Health Nursing, 15*(3), 219–228. https://doi.org/10.1111/j.1365-2850.2007.01215.x

Scott, S., & McManus, S. (2016). *Hidden hurt: Violence, abuse and disadvantage in the lives of women*. Agenda Alliance. https://www.agendaalliance.org/documents/124/Hidden-Hurt-Full-Report.pdf

Scott, E. M., Hermens, D. F., Glozier, N., Naismith, S. L., Guastella, A. J., & Hickie, I. B. (2012). Targeted primary care-based mental health services for young Australians. *Medical Journal of Australia, 196*(2), 136–140. https://doi.org/10.5694/mja11.10481

Scull, A. (2009). *Hysteria: The disturbing history*. OUP.

Scull, A. (2015). *Madness in civilization: A cultural history of insanity, from the bible to Freud, from the madhouse to modern medicine*. Princeton University Press.

Shaw, C., & Proctor, G. (2005). I. Women at the margins: A critique of the diagnosis of borderline personality disorder. *Feminism & Psychology, 15*(4), 483–490.

Showalter, E. (1993). Hysteria, feminism, and gender. In S. L. Gilman, H. King, R. Porter, G. S. Rousseau, & E. Showalter (Eds.), *Hysteria beyond Freud* (pp. 286–344). University of California Press.

de Silva de Alwis, R. (2012). Domestic violence lawmaking in Asia: Some innovative trends in feminist lawmaking. *UCLA Pacific Basin Law Journal, 29*(2), 176. https://doi.org/10.5070/P8292022236

Sinko, L., James, R., & Hughesdon, K. (2022). Healing after gender-based violence: A qualitative meta synthesisusing meta-ethnography. *Trauma, Violence, & Abuse, 23*(4), 1184–1203. https://doi.org/10.1177/1524838021991305

Sinko, L., Dubois, C., & Thorvaldsdottir, K. B. (2024). Measuring healing and recovery after gender-based violence: A scoping review. *Trauma, Violence, & Abuse, 25*(4), 2907–2926.

Smith, M. V., & Mazure, C. M. (2021). Mental health and wealth: Depression, gender, poverty, and parenting. *Annual Review of Clinical Psychology, 17*(1), 181–205. https://doi.org/10.1146/annurev-clinpsy-071219-022710

Sullivan, C., Vaughan, C., & Wright, J. (2020). *Migrant and refugee women's mental health in Australia: A literature review*. School of Population and Global Health, University of Melbourne.

Taylor, J. (2021). *Why women are blamed for everything: Exposing a culture of victim blaming*. Constable.

Taylor, J. (2022). *Sexy but psycho: How the patriarchy uses women's trauma against them*. Little, Brown.

Testa, R. J., Michaels, M. S., Bliss, W., Rogers, M. L., Balsam, K. F., & Joiner, T. (2017). Suicidal ideation in transgender people: Gender minority stress and interpersonal theory factors. *Journal of Abnormal Psychology, 126*(1), 125.

Thompson, L. (2012). *The wandering womb: A cultural history of outrageous beliefs about women*. Prometheus Books.

Tseris, E. (2016). Thinking critically about 'mental health issues' affecting women during/after violence. *Social Alternatives, 35*(4), 37–42.

Tseris, E. (2023). Placing women's mental health in context: The value of a feminist paradigm. *Australian Journal of General Practice, 52*(7) https://www1.racgp.org.au/ajgp/2023/july/placing-womens-mental-health-in-context

Tseris, E. (2024). The myth of trauma-informed mental health services. In C. Brown (Ed.), *Reframing trauma through social justice* (pp. 57–70). Routledge.

Tseris, E., Franks, S., & Hart, E. B. (2024). Benevolence and expertise? Questioning the role of coercive psychiatry in women's lives. In *Psychiatric oppression in women's lives: Creative resistance and collective dissent* (pp. 1–37). Springer International Publishing.

Ussher, J. M. (1991). *Women's madness: Misogyny or mental illness?* University of Massachusetts Press.

Ussher, J. M. (2011). *The madness of women: Myth and experience*. Routledge.

Vranda, M., Janardhana, N., & Kumar, C. (2023). Development of preparedness to respond to intimate partner violence scale among mental health professionals. *Journal of Neurosciences in Rural Practice, 14*(1), 98–102. https://doi.org/10.25259/jnrp-2022-4-31

Walby, S., & Allen, J. (2004). *Domestic violence, sexual assault and stalking: Findings from the British crime survey*. Home Office. https://openaccess.city.ac.uk/id/eprint/21697/1/Domesticviolencefindings_2004_5BritishCrimeSurvey276.pdf

Walby, S., & Towers, J. (2018). Untangling the concept of coercive control: Theorizing domestic violent crime. *Criminology & Criminal Justice, 18*(1), 7–28. https://doi.org/10.1177/1748895817743541

White, S. J., Sin, J., Sweeney, A., Salisbury, T., Wahlich, C., Montesinos Guevara, C. M., et al. (2024). Global prevalence and mental health outcomes of intimate partner violence among women: A systematic review and meta-analysis. *Trauma, Violence, & Abuse, 25*(1), 494–511. https://doi.org/10.1186/s12905-023-02845-8

Wiener, C. (2022). *Coercive control and the criminal law*. Routledge.

Wilkins, R., Laß, I., Butterworth, P., & Vera-Toscano, E. (2019). *The household, income and labour dynamics in Australia survey: Selected findings from waves 1 to 17. The 14th annual statistical report of the HILDA survey.* Melbourne Institute: Applied Economic & Social Research, The University of Melbourne.

Winchester, L. B., Jones, S. C., Allen, K., Hope, E., & Cryer-Coupet, Q. R. (2022). Let's talk: The impact of gendered racial socialization on black adolescent girls' mental health. *Cultural Diversity & Ethnic Minority Psychology, 28*(2), 171.

Wirth-Cauchon, J. (2001). *Women and borderline personality disorder: Symptoms and stories.* Rutgers University Press.

Workplace Gender Equality Agency. (2024). *Gender pay gap data.* Australian Government.https://www.wgea.gov.au/pay-and-gender/gender-pay-gap-data#what-about-the-abs-

World Health Organization (WHO). (2011). *Evidence for gender responsive actions to promote mental health: Young people's health as a whole-of-society response.* WHO Regional Office for Europe.

World Health Organization (WHO). (2020). *Gender and women's mental health.* World Health Organization.

World Health Organization (WHO). (2024). *Violence against women.* https://www.who.int/news-room/fact-sheets/detail/violence-against-women

Zirnsak, T., Elwyn, R., McLoughlan, G., Le Couteur, E., Green, C., Hill, N., Roberts, R., & Maylea, C. (2024). "I have to fight for them to investigate things": A qualitative exploration of physical and mental healthcare for women diagnosed with mental illness. *Frontiers in Public Health, 12*, 1360561.

CHAPTER 3

Peer Support in Mental Health

Michele Jarldorn, Nicole Moulding, and Kate Deuter

Abstract This chapter explores the evolution of peer support in mental health care, tracing its roots in the rights movements of the 1960s and 1970s. The chapter also engages with the emergence of the recovery model of mental health that has arisen hand in hand with the more recent upsurge of interest in peer support in mental health care, highlighting how this has often been associated with treatment in tertiary mental healthcare settings. Lastly, we point to the potential of this approach in feminist approaches to primary mental health care for young women.

Keywords Recovery • Peer support • Feminist social movements • Mental health

M. Jarldorn (✉) · N. Moulding · K. Deuter
University of South Australia, Magill, SA, Australia
e-mail: Michele.jarldorn@unisa.edu.au;
Nicole.Moulding@unisa.edu.au; Kate.Deuter@unisa.edu.au

M. Jarldorn et al. (eds.), *Feminist Action Research in Mental Health*, https://doi.org/10.1007/978-3-032-04406-8_3

Introduction

Individuals have long supported each other informally in the community through mental health self-help groups (Basset et al., 2010; Billsborough et al., 2017) and the practice of mutual aid (Muskat et al., 2020; Rosenwald & Baird, 2020; Spade, 2020). Contemporary models of peer support originated in grassroots, bottom-up movements in mental health and disability rights in western countries in the 1960s and 1970s. In the 2000s, the concept and practice of peer support received increasing attention with the growth in the recovery model of mental health care, particularly its potential in tertiary mental health settings. In this chapter, we chart the history of the emergence of peer support and explore what might be drawn from these models for feminist-informed peer support approaches with young women.

Social Movements and Peer Support

The social rights movements of the 1960s and 1970s pushed for increased involvement of individuals with mental health problems in their own care and were crucial in advancing the peer support agenda (Basset et al., 2010; Billsborough et al., 2017; Faulkner & Kalathil, 2012). These consumer-led movements have driven an increase in user involvement in mental health services, especially since the 1970s (Pitt et al., 2013; Scott et al., 2011; Wright-Berryman et al., 2011). These models take a socio-political focus that "rejects the medical model's discourse and seeks to reconnect individual psychological suffering with social, political, economic, and environmental conditions of oppression and injustice" (Adame & Leitner, 2008, p. 148). As Meadows et al. (2020) explain:

> The mental health consumer movement continues to be an active force in offering an alternative and provocative (re)conceptualisation of mental disorder, in particular the concept of 'consumer perspective', which, like feminism in the 1970s, intimates the possibility of paradigm change in the way in which mental disorder is understood, and service provision shaped or even revolutionised in response to consumer advocacy and participation. (p. 8)

Peer support has been defined as "a system of giving and receiving help founded on key principles of respect, shared responsibility, and mutual agreement of what is helpful" (Mead et al., 2001, p. 135). Hence, peer support is not about people with lived experience of mental illness simply supporting individuals with similar experiences (Adame & Leitner, 2008; Shalaby & Agyapong, 2020). Instead, a recovery-oriented focus in peer support can build on the strength of relationships and community in ways that take into account the social context of mental health problems (Bland et al., 2015).

Some go further and describe the idea of recovery, and the peer support it involves, as a political response to the dehumanisation people have experienced when using mainstream mental health systems (Deegan, 1996; Taylor, 2021). Founded on notions of hope and healing, positive identity, taking responsibility, control and choice, recovery-oriented approaches to mental illness focus on the process and the journey taken by a person as they address the challenges posed by their mental illness, rather than necessarily seeking a cure (Elias & Upton-Davis, 2015). Recovery approaches are also presented as a "synthesis of professional and lived experience" (Glover, 2005, p. 2), informed by the stories of people who have lived with the struggles of mental illness. Within the recovery approach, peers are particularly important because of their capacity to deeply understand what it means to feel powerless within mental health systems, their intimate knowledge of stigma and discrimination and their ability to help others based upon their lived experience (Adame & Leitner, 2008; Davidson et al., 1999; Deegan, 1996).

Peer support approaches to mental health are intrinsically based on principles of respect, shared responsibility and the belief that significant interpersonal relationships and a shared sense of community lay the foundation for recovery (Bland et al., 2015). The approach has been widely supported by practitioners in social work, nursing, and psychology who are involved in the provision of mental health services in Australia and other countries, and is valued due to its emphasis on working with people's strengths (Bland et al., 2015). Roberts and Wolfson (2004) argue that 'narratives of recovery' normalise shared experience and reduce the stigma of mental illness, with peer workers sharing experiences and helpful strategies with individuals experiencing mental health problems while demonstrating a positive example of the potential for recovery can provide hope for the future. Peer support is presented as so central to the recovery approach to mental health care that many see it as exemplifying the approach (e.g., see Slade, 2009). As pointed out in previous chapters, our research was primarily interested in the scope of peer support for young women experiencing common mental health problems such as anxiety, depression and post-traumatic stress disorder. Much of the existing research into peer support focuses on its use with individuals who have serious mental health problems in tertiary care settings, but it is useful to touch briefly on its history in these settings to draw out useful insights for its application in primary healthcare settings.

Peer Support in Psychiatric Settings

Since the middle of the twentieth century, psychiatric in-patient hospitals and units have offered group-based therapy as an extension of individual psychiatric care. Research into peer support work suggests it has a positive impact on service users, as well as on the peer support workers themselves and the healthcare system as a whole (Shalaby & Agyapong, 2020); for example, studies show reduced hospital admissions (Bellamy et al., 2017; Lawn et al., 2008; Lloyd-Evans et al., 2014; Simpson & House, 2002), improved quality of life indicators (Bellamy et al., 2017), a decrease in substance misuse (Davidson et al., 2012) and increased levels of community engagement and inclusion (Bellamy et al., 2017). Because of its relational nature, peer support is thought to improve individual wellbeing by decreasing social isolation and loneliness, thereby supporting individuals in better managing their own mental health (Repper & Carter, 2011). Specifically, the evidence suggests that community-based peer support can provide accessible help outside healthcare services and focus on tailored, relationship-based approaches.

What community-based peer support appears to achieve more successfully than professionally qualified staff is promote hope and belief in the possibility of recovery (Davidson et al., 2012; Repper & Carter, 2011; Seebohm et al., 2013; Siskind et al., 2012). This includes providing individuals with a greater sense of empowerment and increased self-esteem, self-efficacy, social inclusion, engagement and expanded social networks. It has been argued that one of the key benefits of peer support work is not only the worker's familiarity with the symptoms of mental illness, but their understanding of the impact of stigma, stereotyping and social isolation that accompany mental illness and their knowledge of how to navigate complex mental health service systems. Combined with the protective factors of having one's emotional and material needs met (WHO, 2020), peer support is arguably a significant and valuable resource for individuals living with mental health problems. The research demonstrates that, particularly in a group setting, peers can provide significant empathetic support, because the sharing of experiences helps group members to "replace pathological explanations of their situation with more positive interpretations which consider a wider context" (Seebohm et al., 2013, p. 392). Two reports from Australia (Childs, 2021; Gallagher & Halpin, 2014) and one from Scotland (Collumb et al., 2013) also pointed to improvements in individual clients' sense of hope for recovery, self-esteem, decision-making skills including identifying individual coping strategies and managing symptoms, lower rates of isolation, decreased psychiatric symptoms, greater pursuit of educational goals and employment, and a reduction in the impact of stigma. However, although formal peer to peer work in psychiatric settings is very useful for people using services, it can carry challenges for the peer support workers themselves. For example, in a qualitative study of peer mental health workers in the United States, (Moran et al., 2013), peer workers described multiple difficulties that came with their role including lack of training, unclear job descriptions, the physical and emotional impact of high workloads, and struggles when their own symptoms escalated. They also spoke of the distress they felt when co-workers 'vented' and used 'derogatory language' about service users, and their frustration at the realisation that their service did not always follow a recovery-oriented approach, despite claims that they did. Similarly, peer mental health workers in a study by Kemp and Henderson (2012) explained that their main challenge was feeling a sense of exclusion among their colleagues due to a lack of understanding of their roles within their organisation.

While evidence for the benefits of peer support work is strong, much of this research focuses on non-reciprocal relationships in tertiary mental health settings, where the worker is employed because they are at a more 'advanced' stage of recovery into a role that is 'professionalised' (Chinman et al., 2014). Rarely has research explored a mutual horizontal version of peer support where people with a mental illness support each other equally (e.g., Mead & Hilton, 2003; Mead et al., 2001; Pistrang et al., 2008). Moreover, while demonstrating benefits, the peer support programs that are the focus of most research to date have not been gender specific in their orientation, taking a gender neutral approach that does not engage with questions of gender inequality, intersectionality, gendered violence or other forms of gender oppression.

Feminist Approaches to Peer Support

During the 1960s and 1970s, when the consumer-led mental health and disability rights movements began challenging medical dominance, the second wave feminist movement in Australia and many other countries also became active in bringing new understandings of the nature of women's specific struggles with mental health and their basis in gender inequality and gendered violence (Breckenridge & Laing, 1999). The women's movement made enormous use of 'consciousness-raising' and group work, both for political activism but also as a way of providing support for women experiencing gendered violence and for those struggling with mental health (Bondi & Burman, 2001). The approaches deployed by women's groups were based on egalitarian relationships and actively avoided pathologising, deficit-based models when addressing women's mental health concerns (Bondi & Burman, 2001). These groups located women's mental health challenges in the context of the overlapping oppressions of gender, class and race (Waterhouse, 1993; Wright, 2009, pp. 74–75) and, unlike traditional psycho-medical approaches, acknowledged the significant impact of gendered violence on women's health and wellbeing. Many feminist mental health workers and researchers were (and continue to be) involved in challenging psycho-medical approaches to women's mental health and acknowledge the central role of gendered violence in women's distress (Moulding, 2016; Taylor, 2021). While feminist understandings and approaches have been ground-breaking and highly effective, the late 1980s and early 1990s saw a backlash against feminism that sought to reinscribe socially constructed, gendered expectations of women (and men) (Faludi, 2006). This backlash was matched by a burgeoning of neoliberal ideals of individual responsibility in which mental health support became the domain of professional experts in clinical, one-on-one settings (Timler, 2022; Bondi & Burman, 2001). As Bondi and Burman (2001) explain, professionals tend to convey "normative conceptions of gender and sexuality" (p. 17) and are therefore unlikely to consider the role of gendered violence as the underlying cause of mental distress. They are also unlikely to look to other forms of gender inequality that impact on women's lives.

While a feminist approach to women's mental health care that places experience in its gendered social context has been the subject of extensive feminist advocacy and activism from the 1970s to the present day, this has been slow to translate into mental health policy (O'Connor et al., 2025), where representations of women in Australian mental health policy are underpinned by biomedical and neoliberal thinking (O'Connor et al., 2025). Biomedical discourse locates women's mental distress within their physical selves and supports a medicalised approach involving diagnosis, the use of medication and other psychiatric interventions. Similarly, neoliberal discourses place responsibility on the failed neoliberal subject for their distress, usually for their 'poor choices', and the need for individuals to take responsibility for themselves by managing risk and making themselves 'better'. These discourses are steeped in gendered assumptions and stereotypes and are woven throughout mental health policies in Australia. As O'Connor et al. (2025) argue, "policy is not politically or socially neutral because it is created in a social context of contested discourses" (p. 73) and in doing so, they can successfully shift the focus away from the need for structural and cultural change, improved social conditions or increased gender equity and equality.

Over recent decades, there have been many attempts to set out what positive, socially informed feminist mental health policy and service provision would look like. Some of the recommendations have included the provision of gender-sensitive mental health supports, including the formation of women-only services that use a trauma-informed approach, and ensuring workers' caseloads provide service users with the space and time to talk to women and provide choices for their care using a life-stage approach (Newbigging & Abel, 2006; Tseris, 2024). Other suggestions include the need to pay attention to the individual factors in women's lives in concert with the socio-cultural and structural contexts they live in. Such models of service provision use an intersectional approach, provide holistic, strengths-based approaches to women's mental health challenges (Agenda & AVA, 2019: 11–12), encourage women to support each other, be active participants in their own care (Chandra et al., 2019, p. 760) and approach support as "a dialogue between equals" (Payne, 2017, p. 29). Importantly, feminist informed approaches take into consideration "women's intersecting experiences of mental ill health, homelessness, substance misuse, poverty, violence and contact with the criminal justice system" (Andleeb et al., 2020, p. 11) as well as experiences relating to race, ethnicity, immigration status, sexuality, socio-economic position and living with disability (Agenda & AVA, 2019).

In view of the gender inequalities outlined in the previous chapter, it is clear that young women's experiences of diagnosis, their lived experience of the mental health problem itself, and their recovery experiences, are significantly different to those of men. As a result of these distinctive features in young women's mental health journeys, policies and strategies to facilitate and support young women to maintain social connectivity and manage good mental health and wellbeing outside of traditional mental health services and facilities are critical (Bäckström Olofsson & Goicolea, 2024; Bäckström Olofsson, 2025; Maidment et al., 2024; O'Connor et al., 2025; Pound et al., 2011). Peer support is one such strategy that can provide an important vehicle for the realisation of recovery (Collaton et al., 2022; Lawn et al., 2008).

Supportive connections between peers can centre individual empowerment and healing (McColl et al., 2014), acknowledging the diverse social contexts in which they live, the significant interpersonal relationships in their lives and the importance of a shared sense of community as integral to recovery (Pound et al., 2011). A peer support approach informed by a social perspective on young women's mental health can therefore offer safe spaces in which young women can flourish both personally and socially.

There is evidence that gender-aware approaches to primary mental health peer support are effective (Andleeb et al., 2020; Bäckström Olofsson & Goicolea, 2024), with significant unmet demand for this type of approach. For example, results from a global survey exploring the integration of gender into mental health services, Chandra et al. (2019) found that while the majority of mental health professionals agreed with the need for services to be gender sensitive, there was little evidence to support that this awareness translated into action. So, while the evidence supporting the efficacy of gender-responsive peer led services exists, particularly for using collaborative and clearly articulated feminist principles (see, e.g., Bäckström Olofsson & Goicolea, 2024), there has been limited effort to develop such approaches more broadly in policy and practice.

Feminist approaches to the provision of support to young women is not simply a matter of choice and preference; such approaches can provide space and support that recognises and address trauma in ways that are not undertaken by services that are blind to the gendered nature of young women's experiences and needs (Agenda & AVA, 2019). Specifically, trauma-informed, gender-responsive peer support has been shown to increase social networks and self-esteem among women, including young women, both of which are indicators of improved mental wellbeing (Andleeb et al., 2020). In line with findings reported by AVA and Agenda (2017), gender-responsive peer support for young women also has a measurable positive impact on a range of other outcomes that are linked to improved wellbeing, revealing that the way support is provided can make important differences to outcomes. As Gillard (2019) points out:

> A strong argument can be made…that peer support might be better situated outside of the constraining culture of formal mental health services (and that as researchers we might therefore better focus on evaluating those endeavours) (p. 342)

This suggests that peer designed, informed and driven supports for the mental wellbeing of young women should be led by young women themselves, with a role for skilled practitioners to work alongside them to support them in the development of peer support opportunities. Such efforts could draw on co-design principles and an egalitarian approach to whose knowledge is privileged, offering possibilities for the development of alternative approaches to promoting wellbeing for young women. The provision of a critical feminist approach to supporting young women's mental wellbeing would help to ensure their struggles are understood as located in gendered historical, symbolic, structural and systemic oppressions that intersect with racism, colonialism, ableism, transphobia and homophobia.

While there has been a relative lack of attention in research and practice to the social contexts in which mental health problems develop, there has been a growing understanding over the past decade of the need to consider and respond to previous experiences of trauma when working alongside people accessing social and health services. Often called 'trauma-informed practice', this approach seeks to engage with individual trauma histories and their role in poor mental health (Kezelman & Stavropoulos, 2012) and avoids blaming or excluding individuals for coping mechanisms that arise from negative life experiences (Levenson, 2017). Evidence suggests that taking past experiences of trauma into account in peer-to-peer mental health can be effective (Elliott et al., 2005; Gillard, 2019; Hopper et al., 2010). However, the term 'trauma-informed' has become co-opted and mainstreamed to the point where it has become over-used with minimal guidance on how to enact it in practice (Tseris, 2024). Additionally, while being 'trauma-informed' is important for its acknowledgement of the impact of interpersonal violence and abuse on mental health, like other mainstream mental health practices in Australia, current models take a largely gender-blind and gender-neutral approach (Moulding et al., 2021).

At this point, it is useful to offer an illustration from our own research which shows how feminist trauma-informed peer support can be radically different to the type of mental health care women commonly receive in mainstream services. A few years ago, one of us conducted with other colleagues a large Australian research study into the impact of intimate partner violence on women's lives, including on their mental health and wellbeing (Franzway et al., 2018; Moulding et al., 2021). A large sample of women—659—participated in the study. The study found that less than 14% had experienced mental health problems *prior* to living with a violent partner, but that 90% struggled with mental health *during* domestic violence and 65% continued to struggle with their mental health *after they left* (Franzway et al., 2018; Moulding et al., 2021). Many women spoke of the difficulties they experienced in accessing effective mental health care that took into account their experiences of gendered violence. One woman explained her experiences in a particularly evocative way:

> All GPs will do is just put you on anti-depressants which don't work. The issue isn't the chemicals in my brain. The issue is my life sucks … circumstantial depression isn't
>
> best treated by anti-depressants, anti-depressants are for … stabilisation for chemical imbalances, it's not the right treatment, but it's all a GP can offer.

Other women were similarly critical of medicalised approaches to the distress they were experiencing as a result of gendered violence. By way of contrast, women also offered insights into their experiences of peer support in women's groups.

> I was regularly going to the women's group and without that support I would not have gotten through this with no doubt about it at all, I had a whole network of people
>
> helping me to get rid of him … I needed to go to that women's group because that was the only way I could make sense of it all. Once I started hearing all these stories
>
> about how all these other people had been in the same situation …[.]….I needed all this ongoing support … they had a "sister system" … [it] made all the difference.

The above account points to the importance of discovering that other women had very similar experiences and how, as a group, they could support each other in ways that mainstream services could not (Franzway et al., 2018; Moulding et al., 2021).

Conclusion

In this chapter, we have explained how peer support can work as a distinctive approach to mental health care that differs in many important respects from professional care. In so doing, we have shown that most peer support work to date has been gender-blind and undertaken in psychiatric settings. Instead, we have argued for peer support that is gender aware and trauma-informed, and that brings an intersectional lens to understanding and responding to women's struggles around mental health and wellbeing. It is clear from the evidence that feminist models of peer support for young women can bring many benefits that are distinctive to those offered by practitioners. While we have been critical of the pathologisation, individualism and lack of gender awareness that can haunt traditional mental health care, we are not suggesting that mainstream service provision has no role to play if it is gender and trauma aware. However, peer support can offer benefits that are qualitatively distinct from professional support because experiences are shared, power relations between helped and helper are more equal, and there are enhanced opportunities for making connections between women's individual lived experiences and the social structures and cultural norms that frame and shape them. In the following chapter, we explore the benefits of using feminist theory to shape and inform social research into young women's mental health and wellbeing.

References

Adame, A. L., & Leitner, L. M. (2008). Breaking out of the mainstream: The evolution of peer support alternatives to the mental health system. *Ethical Human Psychology and Psychiatry, 10*(3), 146–162. https://doi.org/10.1891/1559-4343.10.3.146

Agenda & AVA. (2019). *Breaking down the barriers: Findings of the national commission on domestic and sexual violence and multiple disadvantage*. https://weareagenda.org/wp-content/uploads/2019/02/Breakingdown-the-Barriers-full-report-FINAL.pdf

Andleeb, H., Parker, J., Mackay, T., Matthews, F., McWilliam, J., Haider, F., Iqbal, N., White, S., & Pinfold, V. (2020). *Evaluation of the women side by side project. Final report.* McPin Foundation and St George's University of London, UK.

AVA, & Agenda. (2017). *Mapping the Maze: Services for women experiencing multiple disadvantages in England and Wales.* https://www.mappingthemaze.org.uk/wp/wp-content/uploads/2017/02/Mapping-the-Mazefinal-report-for-publication.pdf

Bäckström Olofsson, H. (2025). "Being a girl has become a public health problem!": Feminist organizations both resisting and reproducing postfeminist mental health discourses. *NORA-Nordic Journal of Feminist and Gender Research, 33*(1), 31–44. https://doi.org/10.1080/08038740.2024.2354770

Bäckström Olofsson, H., & Goicolea, I. (2024). Sisterhood at a distance: Doing feminist support work online. *Affilia, 39*(2), 214–228. https://doi.org/10.1177/08861099231181583

Basset, T., Faulkner, A., Repper, J., & Stamou, E. (2010). *Lived experience leading the way peer support in mental health.* University of Nottingham.

Bellamy, C., Schmutte, T., & Davidson, L. (2017). An update on the growing evidence base for peer support. *Mental Health and Social Inclusion, 21*(3), 161–167. https://doi.org/10.1108/MHSI-03-2017-0014

Billsborough, J., Currie, Gibson, Gillard, S., Golightley, S., Kotecha-Hazzard, R., Mesaric, A., Mohammed, S., Pinfold, V., Sweet, D., Thompson, R., & White, S. (2017). *Evaluating the side by side peer support programme.* McPin Foundation and St George's University of London.

Bland, R., Renouf, N., & Tullgren, A. (2015). *Social work practice in mental health: An introduction* (2nd ed.). Allen & Unwin.

Bondi, L., & Burman, E. (2001). Women and mental health: A feminist review. *Feminist Review, 68*(1), 6–33. https://doi.org/10.1080/01417780122133

Breckenridge, J., & Laing, L. (1999). *Challenging silence: Innovative responses to sexual and domestic violence.* Allen & Unwin.

Chandra, P. S., Saraf, G., Bajaj, A., & Satyanarayana, V. A. (2019). The current status of gender-sensitive mental health services for women—Findings from a global survey of experts. *Archives of Women's Mental Health, 22*(6), 759–770. https://doi.org/10.1007/s00737-019-01001-2

Childs, B. (2021). *Mind's peer work framework.* https://www.mindaustralia.org.au/work-us/peer-work

Chinman, M., George, P., Dougherty, R. H., Daniels, A. S., Ghose, S. S., Swift, A., & Delphin-Rittmon, M. E. (2014). Peer support services for individuals with serious mental illnesses: Assessing the evidence. *Psychiatric Services, 65*(4), 429–441. https://doi.org/10.1176/appi.ps.201300244

Collaton, J., Barata, P., & Lewis, S. P. (2022). Understanding discussions of sexual assault in young women on a peer support mental health app: A content analysis. *Journal of Interpersonal Violence, 37*(23–24), NP22811–NP22833. https://doi.org/10.21428/cb6ab371.91f6e634

Collumb, S., Gillespie, M., Grant, G., Hansen, D., Kernohan, A., Lear, S., McBrierty, R., Nicholson, J., & Pollock, S. (2013). *Values framework for peer learning*. https://mhcsa.org.au/wpcontent/uploads/2021/09/SRN_Values_Framework_Peer_Working_reprint_2013.pdf

Davidson, L., Chinman, M., Kloos, B., Weingarten, R., Stayner, D., & Kraemer Tebes, J. (1999). Peer support among individuals with severe mental illness: A review of the evidence. *Clinical Psychology: Science and Practice, 6*(2), 165. https://doi.org/10.1093/clipsy.6.2.165

Davidson, L., Bellamy, C., Guy, K., & Miller, R. (2012). Peer support among individuals with severe mental illness: A review of the evidence and experience. *World Psychiatry, 11*(2), 123–128. https://doi.org/10.1016/j.wpsyc.2012.05.009

Deegan, P. (1996). Recovery as a journey of the heart. *Psychiatric Rehabilitation Journal, 19*(3), 91–97. https://psycnet.apa.org/doi/10.1037/h0101301

Elias, P., & Upton-Davis, K. (2015). Embedding peer support using social work values. *The Journal of Mental Health Training, Education, and Practice, 10*(5), 304–313. https://doi.org/10.1108/JMHTEP-06-2015-0028

Elliott, D. E., Bjelajac, P., Fallot, R. D., Markoff, L. S., & Reed, B. G. (2005). Trauma-informed or trauma-denied: Principles and implementation of trauma-informed services for women. *Journal of Community Psychology, 33*(4), 461–477. https://doi.org/10.1002/jcop.20063

Faludi, S. (2006). *Backlash: The undeclared war against American women*. Crown Publishing Group.

Faulkner, A., & Kalathil, J. (2012). *The freedom to be, the chance to dream: Preserving user-led peer support in mental health*. https://www.together-uk.org/wp-content/uploads/2012/09/The-Freedom-to-be-The-Chance-to-dream-Full-Report1.pdf

Franzway, S., Moulding, N., Wendt, S., Zufferey, C., & Chung, D. (2018). *The sexual politics of gendered violence and women's citizenship*. Policy Press. https://doi.org/10.1332/policypress/9781447337782.003.0001

Gallagher, C., & Halpin, M. (2014). *The lived experience workforce in South Australian public mental health services: What we have learned, what we have achieved and future directions*. https://mhcsa.org.au/wp-content/uploads/2021/09/The-Lived-Experience-Workforce-in-SA-Public-Mental-Health-Services.pdf

Gillard, S. (2019). Peer support in mental health services: Where is the research taking us, and do we want to go there? *Journal of Mental Health, 28*(4), 341–344. https://doi.org/10.1080/09638237.2019.1608935

Glover, H. (2005). Recovery based service delivery: Are we ready to transform the words into a paradigm shift? *Australian e-Journal for the Advancement of Mental Health, 4*(3), 179–182. https://doi.org/10.5172/jamh.4.3.179

Hopper, E. K., Bassuk, E. L., & Olivet, J. (2010). Shelter from the storm: Trauma-informed care in homelessness services settings. *The Open Health*

Services and Policy Journal, 3(1), 80–100. http://dx.doi.org/%20 10.2174/1874924001003010080

Kemp, V., & Henderson, A. R. (2012). Challenges faced by mental health peer support workers: Peer support from the peer supporter's point of view. *Psychiatric Rehabilitation Journal, 35*(4), 337–340. https://doi.org/10.2975/35.4.2012.337.340

Kezelman, C., & Stavropoulos, P. (2012). Practice guidelines for treatment of complex trauma and trauma informed care and service delivery. *Sydney: Adults Surviving Child Abuse.* https://www.childabuseroyalcommission.gov.au/sites/default/files/IND.0521.001.0001.pdf

Lawn, S., Smith, A., & Hunter, K. (2008). Mental health peer support for hospital avoidance and early discharge: An Australian example of consumer-driven and operated service. *Journal of Mental Health, 17*(5), 498–508. https://doi.org/10.1080/09638230701530242

Levenson, J. (2017). Trauma informed social work practice. *Social Work, 62*(2), 105–113. https://doi.org/10.1093/sw/swx001

Lloyd-Evans, B., Mayo-Wilson, E., Harrison, B., Istead, H., Brown, E., Pilling, S., Johnson, S., & Kendall, T. (2014). A systematic review and meta-analysis of randomised controlled trials of peer support for people with severe mental illness. *BMC Psychiatry, 14*(1), 39–39. https://doi.org/10.1186/1471-244X-14-39

Maidment, K., Jenkins, K., Houlihan, M. & the Prevention United Youth Advisory Group (YAG). (2024). *Policy Brief: The significance of gender-based violence as a key driver in young women's disproportionate experiences of mental ill-health* Prevention United, Melbourne. https://anrows.intersearch.com.au/anrowsjspui/bitstream/1/22787/1/apo-nid328294.pdf

McColl, L. D., Rideout, P. E., Parmar, T. N., & Abba-Aji, A. (2014). Peer support intervention through Mobile application: An integrative literature review and future directions. *Canadian Psychology (Psychologie Canadienne), 55*(4), 250–257.

Mead, S., & Hilton, D. (2003). Crisis and connection. *Psychiatric Rehabilitation Journal, 27*(1), 87–95. https://psycnet.apa.org/doi/10.2975/27.2003.87.94

Mead, S., Hilton, D., & Curtis, L. (2001). Peer-support: A theoretical perspective. *Psychiatric Rehabilitation Journal, 25*(2), 134–141. https://doi.org/10.1037/h0095032

Meadows, G., Farhall, J., Fossey, E., Happell, B., Grigg, M., McDermott, F., Rosenberg, S., & Singh, B. (2020). *Mental health in Australia: Collaborative community practice* (4th ed.). Oxford University Press.

Moran, G. S., Russinova, Z., Gidugu, V., & Gagne, C. (2013). Challenges experienced by paid peer providers in mental health recovery: A qualitative study. *Community Mental Health Journal, 49*(3), 281–291. https://doi.org/10.1007/s10597-012-9541-y

Moulding, N. T. (2016). *Gendered violence, abuse and mental health in everyday lives: Beyond trauma*. Routledge. https://doi.org/10.4324/9781315816630

Moulding, N., Franzway, S., Wendt, S., Zufferey, C., & Chung, D. (2021). Rethinking women's mental health after intimate partner violence. *Violence Against Women, 27*(8), 1064–1090. https://doi.org/10.1177/1077801220921937

Muskat, B., Greenblatt, A., Garvin, C., Pelech, W., Cohen, C., Macgowan, M., & Roy, V. (2020). Group workers' experiences of mutual aid: Stories from the field. *Social Work with Groups (New York. 1978), 43*(3), 241–256. https://doi.org/10.1080/01609513.2019.1571470

Newbigging, K., & Abel, K. (2006). *Supporting women into the mainstream: Commissioning women-only community day services*. Department of Health.

O'Connor, C. A., Zufferey, C., & de Anstiss, H. (2025). Governing failed neoliberal subjects: Representations of women's mental health in Australian mental health policies. *Qualitative Social Work, 24*(1), 61–77. https://doi.org/10.1177/14733250231222020

Payne, M. (2017). Peer support in mental health: A narrative review of its relevance to social work. *The Egyptian Journal of Social Work, 4*(1), 20–40. https://doi.org/10.21608/ejsw.2017.8725

Pistrang, N., Barker, C., & Humphreys, K. (2008). Mutual help groups for mental health problems: A review of effectiveness studies. *American Journal of Community Psychology, 42*(1–2), 110–121. https://doi.org/10.1007/s10464-008-9181-0

Pitt, V., Lowe, D., Hill, S., Prictor, M., Hetrick, S. E., Ryan, R., & Berends, L. (2013). Consumer-providers of care for adult clients of statutory mental health services. Cochrane. *Library, 3*, CD004807. https://doi.org/10.1002/14651858.CD004807.pub2

Pound, L., Judd, K., & Gough, J. (2011). *Peer support for women living with mental health issues: The views of ACT women*. https://www.womenshealthmatters.org.au/wp-content/uploads/2020/10/Peer-support-for-women-with-mental-health-issues-The-views-of-ACT-women.pdf

Repper, J., & Carter, T. (2011). A review of the literature on peer support in mental health services. *Journal of Mental Health, 20*(4), 392–411. https://doi.org/10.3109/09638237.2011.583947

Roberts, G., & Wolfson, P. (2004). The rediscovery of recovery: Open to all. *Advances in Psychiatric Treatment, 10*(1), 37–48. https://doi.org/10.1192/apt.10.1.37

Rosenwald, M., & Baird, J. (2020). An integrated trauma-informed, mutual aid model of group work. *Social Work With Groups, 43*(3), 257–271. https://doi.org/10.1016/j.socscimed.2004.08.026

Scott, A., Doughty, C., & Kahi, H. (2011). *Peer support practice in Aotearoa New Zealand*. University of Canterbury.

Seebohm, P., Chaudhary, S., Boyce, M., Elkan, R., Avis, M., & Munn-Giddings, C. (2013). The contribution of self-help/mutual aid groups to mental well-being. *Health & Social Care in the Community, 21*(4), 391–401. https://doi.org/10.1111/hsc.12021

Shalaby, R. A. H., & Agyapong, V. I. (2020). Peer support in mental health: Literature review. *JMIR Mental Health, 7*(6), e15572. https://doi.org/10.2196/15572

Simpson, E. L., & House, A. O. (2002). Involving users in the delivery and evaluation of mental health services: Systematic review. *BMJ, 325*(7375), 1265–1268. https://doi.org/10.1136/bmj.325.7375.1265

Siskind, D., Harris, M., Pirkis, J., & Whiteford, H. (2012). Personalised support delivered by support workers for people with severe and persistent mental illness: A systematic review of patient outcomes. *Epidemiology and Psychiatric Sciences, 21*(1), 97–110. https://doi.org/10.1017/S2045796011000734

Slade, M. (2009). *Personal recovery and mental illness. A guide for mental health professionals.* Cambridge University Press.

Spade, D. (2020). Solidarity not charity. Mutual aid for mobilization and survival. *Social Text, 38*(1), 131–151. https://doi.org/10.1215/01642472-7971139

Taylor, J. (2021). *Why women are blamed for everything: Exposing a culture of victim blaming.* Constable.

Timler, K. (2022). Distorted thinking or distorted realities? The social construction of anxiety for women in neoliberal late-stage capitalism. *Hypatia, 37*(4), 726–742. https://doi.org/10.1017/hyp.2022.60

Tseris, E. (2024). The myth of trauma-informed mental health services. In C. Brown (Ed.), *Reframing trauma through social justice* (pp. 57–70). Routledge.

Waterhouse, R. L. (1993). 'Wild women don't have the blues': A feminist critique of person-centred counselling and therapy. *Feminism & Psychology, 3*(1), 55–71. https://doi.org/10.1177/0959353593031004

World Health Organization (WHO). (2020). *Gender and women's mental health.* World Health Organization.

Wright, J. (2009). Unfinished business with feminist thinking and counselling and guidance practice. *British Journal of Guidance & Counselling, 37*(1), 73–82. https://doi.org/10.1080/03069880802534088

Wright-Berryman, J. L., McGuire, A. B., & Salyers, M. P. (2011). A review of consumer-provided services on assertive community treatment and intensive case management teams: Implications for future research and practice. *Journal of the American Psychiatric Nurses Association, 17*(1), 37–44. https://doi.org/10.1177/10783903103932

CHAPTER 4

A Feminist Approach to Participatory co-Design Research

Nicole Moulding and Michele Jarldorn

Abstract In this chapter, we familiarise you with the theoretical framework we used to guide our co-designed research project. The approach effectively involved a quilting together of key feminist concepts that explain structural gender inequalities and socio-cultural gender discourses (McNay, L., *The Sociological Review 52*:175-190, 2004), intersectionality (Crenshaw, K., *Stanford Law Review 43*:1241, 1991) and a feminist approach to participatory action research guided by a feminist ethics of care (Miele, R., Root, J., Godderis, R., & Meerai, S., *Studies in Social Justice, 18*(1), 125-142, 2024). The central aim of the chapter is to demonstrate how a feminist perspective can guide the processes of participatory and action-oriented co-design methods in ways that include young women and strive towards increased gender equality in society.

Keywords Feminist research methods • Positionality • Feminist ethics of care • Participatory action research

N. Moulding · M. Jarldorn (✉)
University of South Australia, Magill, SA, Australia
e-mail: Nicole.Moulding@unisa.edu.au; Michele.jarldorn@unisa.edu.au

M. Jarldorn et al. (eds.), *Feminist Action Research in Mental Health*, https://doi.org/10.1007/978-3-032-04406-8_4

Introduction

Feminist research is distinctive for its emphasis on including women's voices based on a recognition that 'the personal is political' (Hanisch, 1970), and for its quest to better understand the gender inequalities that structure every society across the globe (Ackerly & True, 2010). Feminist *action* research seeks to question and actively disrupt deeply rooted and often unseen and unrecognised operations of patriarchal power embedded in institutional, social and economic systems (Frisby et al., 2009, p. 14). However, while these core characteristics unite feminist approaches, there are many different feminisms (see Mackay, 2015) and, by extension, many different approaches to feminist research. In this chapter, we explain why a feminist positionality was important to the co-designed project we undertook with young women. We then outline the specific feminist theoretical framework that informed our thinking, and how this knitted into a feminist co-design research project.

A Feminist Positionality

A feminist 'positionality' in research involves actively and transparently positioning yourself as the researcher. More traditional research presents itself as 'objective' and 'gender-neutral', seeing itself as getting to the core truth of the problems it studies. Feminists, along with many other social scientists, acknowledge that there is no such thing as total objectivity and that researchers are always operating from a 'position' even if they are not aware of it themselves. All researchers bring their own beliefs to the research table, and these are shaped by that individual's personal and professional experiences (Davis & Khonach, 2020; Frisby et al., 2009). For these reasons and more, many feminist scholars have called on all researchers to directly and openly position themselves in their research processes, including in their publications (Jackson et al., 2024). By positioning themselves, feminists have been able to show that much research purporting to be 'gender-neutral' is in fact fundamentally gender-biased in its assumptions about women and men.

The Harms of Gender-Biased Research

Medical research and the wider medical literature are replete with gender-biased assumptions about women and their bodies. The second wave of feminism played a key role in challenging gender-biased assumptions in women's health research and practice—however, three decades later, there is still some way to go to meet gender equity in health care (Meyers-Pantele et al., 2024; Munch, 2004; Thompson & Blake, 2021). Gender bias against women in medicine takes many forms, where the "language and metaphors used in both medical texts and clinical practice describe women's reproductive-related functions in terms of weakness and pathology" (Munch, 2004, p. 102). The readily accepted assumption that women's distress from physical pain and discomfort is 'in their heads' and thus requires a mental health diagnosis has often led to a failure to diagnose life-threatening physical health conditions, especially when connected to women's reproductive health (Lennane & Lennane, 1973). In another example, gendered expectations of behaviour in social settings have contributed to the underdiagnosis of autism in young girls because of the efforts they expend in masking their autistic characteristics (Hamdani et al., 2023). A further illustration of the idea that 'it's all in her head' can be found in the longstanding construction of myalgic encephalomyelitis/chronic fatigue syndrome (ME/CFS)—which is disproportionately experienced by women—as a somatisation disorder arising from psychological distress. This construction is based on gendered views of female distress, foreclosing consideration that the condition might have a biological basis (Komaroff & Lipkin, 2023). Since the COVID pandemic and the emergence of long COVID in many groups in the population, there has been increasing realisation that viruses can indeed cause symptoms like those experienced in ME/CFS (Komaroff & Lipkin, 2023). A final example is the historical construction of women who have experienced child sexual abuse as 'personality disordered', with little attention to their experiences of gendered abuse in a male dominated gender order and how these can lead to particular coping styles (van der Kolk et al., 1994). Each of these examples illustrates in different ways how a masculinist medical worldview has failed to serve women's health by pathologising women's reproductive functions, by relying on male-centred constructions of health problems that overlook the way conditions present differently in women and by constructing physical health problems disproportionately experienced by women as versions of female 'hysteria'.

Yet, while feminists transparently declare a position, somewhat paradoxically, it is we who are often charged with 'bias' and 'self-involvement'. As has been pointed out previously, "It should be noted here that white men, regardless of what they are studying, rarely are viewed as biased researchers engaged in "mesearch" (Davis & Khonach, 2020, p. 109). This has been called the 'paradox of positionality' (Davis & Khonach, 2020, p. 109) in that it is those who have been honest and transparent about where they are coming from who come to be cast as partial, while those who make pretences to objectivity and truth remain strangely untainted.

A feminist positionality affects every step in the research process, from the types of questions asked by the researchers, to how the researchers conduct themselves during the study, to the approaches to data analysis they adopt and the way they write up their findings (Davis & Khonach, 2020; Srivarathan, 2022). In terms of *how* research should be conducted from a feminist position, there is an emphasis on reducing the power differentials between the researcher and the researched, including acknowledging shared experiences and recognising that both researcher and researched are together making new knowledge (Frisby et al., 2009; Mulvey et al., 2000). This egalitarian approach in combination with the use of self, or positionality, should be used to shape and inform critical feminist research and authorship. This enables feminist researchers to "transparently situate, re-imagine, and mobilize transgressive knowledge production and political action" in ways that engage with questions about "the relationships to power in which all claims to knowledge are embedded" (Jackson et al., 2024, pp. 8–9).

The contribution of a feminist positionality to understanding women's lives and responding to the problems women face cannot be underestimated. This approach challenges the traditional sociological position that the male experience is universal (Smith, 1987). As has been pointed out by UK feminist researcher Finn Mackay (2021), there are no responses to sexual violence, domestic abuse and other forms of gender-based violence (GBV) that are not feminist-informed. Mackay points out that laws, policies and services in the domestic violence area are a direct legacy of the work undertaken by feminists in the second wave; the same can be said about Australia. Mackay (2021) goes further, arguing that "without feminist theory, we could not imagine a world without GBV" (p.4) because everything that is known about the everyday forms of violence that women live through derives from feminist social scientists and activists. Although, as Mimi Kim has argued, the ways responses to gendered violence are shaped are borne out of the shifting approaches to feminist thinking, with progressive ideas typically emerging from communities of colour (Kim, 2018, 2020).

A Feminist Theoretical Framework for Researching Young Women's Mental Health

Over recent decades, there has been much debate within feminist circles about how much emphasis should be given to the cultural and discursive aspects of gender oppression, and how much should be given to the material and structural aspects. To make clearer what we mean by these terms, let us give an example from the area of mental health and wellbeing. As noted in the introduction to this chapter, 'the cultural' aspects of gender oppression refer to discourses for post-structural researchers, or gender norms and beliefs to other feminist researchers (McNay, 2004). We prefer the Foucauldian concept of discourse because it recognises that ideas about gender and mental health have long historical roots and are not fixed but fluid and often highly contradictory (Weedon, 1996); concepts such as 'norms' or 'attitudes' tend to oversimplify and imply a level of fixedness and stability that are not borne out when we examine what people actually say and do in everyday life or in public life, either. For example, gendered femininity discourses portray women as naturally more emotional than men, even expecting and requiring women to perform emotion in social situations (Moulding, 2016). When women do not perform emotion as expected, they can be constructed as untrustworthy or devious; the infamous case of Lindy Chamberlain (Middleweek, 2017) is a case in point, whose 'trial by media' was fuelled by gendered bias because she "...didn't cry enough; she failed to scream enough, wail enough or show enough 'feminine' emotion" (Lambert-Patel, 2020, para. 7). This is not an isolated example; many other women are "routinely held to a different standard" (Lambert-Patel, 2020, para. 11) and are vilified in mainstream media for perceived lack of emotion in tragic circumstances. At the same time, though, women are also pathologised through psychiatric discourses for the demonstration of emotional distress. As can be seen, then, women can face a 'damned if she does, damned if she doesn't' scenario around emotionality that reflects their positioning in male dominated societies as both passive and weak, *and* dangerous and in need of control (Taylor, 2021, 2022).

In the area of young women's mental health, the discursive aspects of gender oppression therefore point to the role of gender discourses about inherent female emotionality and mental instability as well as medical discourses about sick female bodies and minds (Moulding, 2016). Working in concert with these ideas are complementary notions that women are biologically suited to caring roles and therefore should be happy in those roles and not experience distress because of them (Moulding, 2016). Other discourses are also relevant to women's mental health, particularly that of young women, such as those in play in relation to the experience of sexual violence, where women are held responsible and blamed for the rapes and sexual assaults they experience (Gavey, 2005).

Intertwined with the gender and medical discourses that steep and shape women's mental health experiences are the material inequalities inherent within the hierarchical gender order (McNay, 2004). The organisation of patriarchal society and the gender roles and relations that are part and parcel of it mean that most women have less power than men in many life domains, public and private (McNay, 2004). The most fundamental divide here is that between the public and private spheres, with women historically located in the latter (Franzway, 2016). While there has been much change over the past 50 years, vicissitudes of this divide remain and continue to impact on women in a multitude of ways. These include the gender pay gap (Risse, 2024), the lack of access to affordable childcare (Jenkins, 2021) and the over-representation of men in parliament and in all decision-making bodies throughout society (Brown, 2024). Women are also concentrated in low pay, lower status 'caring' occupations, carry a higher burden of domestic and care work and are over-represented on benefits and among those living in poverty (Westmore, 2024). These experiences have a multiplier effect that reach into later life, where women have lower levels of adequate superannuation in old age, lower homeownership rates and poorer health outcomes (Franzway et al., 2019; Macdonald, 2024). These inequalities shape and are shaped by inappropriate social policy and lack of service provision (Maclean & Groves, 2024), leading to inadequate sexual healthcare services, underfunded domestic violence services and, more recently, a revitalised push to reduce women's bodily autonomy through the restriction of reproductive rights. This persistent gender inequality is one of the most common and widespread forms of social inequality in the world, occurring in both private and public spheres (Oxfam, n.d.). All of these factors play a compounding role in women's mental health and wellbeing that persist across the life course.

The feminist approach we adopted for this project takes the view that the cultural and discursive aspects of gender oppression, and the material and structural elements, are equally important, intrinsically tied to each other and reinforce each other (McNay, 2004). Using one of the earlier examples, then, the historical material and structural arrangements that have located women primarily in the home are underpinned and reinforced by discourses about the supposed naturalness and biological basis of these arrangements. When women struggle with postnatal depression as stay at home mothers no longer participating in the paid workforce (a structural arrangement), they often sense that they should not feel the way they do and others around them, including healthcare providers, can reinforce this by mobilising discourses about mothering and care work as 'natural' for women (a gendered socio-cultural discourse) (Moulding, 2019; Zufferey & Buchanan, 2019). The risk of domestic violence and the mental health problems that occur because of this are further heightened when women become financially dependent as stay at home mothers (Stewart, 2021). Here, the new structural arrangement works hand in hand with discourses about the naturalness of these arrangements along with ideas about women and children as the property of male 'heads' of families and primary breadwinners. Here, then, the material and the discursive are clearly and closely entwined and work in concert with one another.

Using an Intersectional Lens

Researching women's experiences must be informed by a multidimensional intersectional framework that "focus[es] on how oppressions of race and gender intersect as mutually constructing systems of power" (Zufferey & Buchanan, 2019, p. 4). Our approach was framed by a contemporary feminist understanding that race, class, age, ableism and sexuality intersect with experiences of gender inequality and oppression in complex ways (Crenshaw, 1991). We understand that "…intersectionality and positionality orient the question of difference, knowledge and power towards action" (Peake & Sharp, 2024, p. 122). However, we also understand gender oppression to be a phenomenon in its own right that has implications for women's experiences across the board, which are then complicated and exacerbated by intersectional inequalities and identities. While we have mapped out our feminist perspective in undertaking research and co-design focused on young women's mental health, perhaps the most important aspect of our approach is the understanding that change is possible and that the discourses and material structural arrangements that underscore women's mental health and wellbeing are not fixed and immutable but open to contestation and change (McNay, 2004). Such change can be actualised by bringing an intersectional focus to the mental health service needs of young women through a women-centred mental healthcare model that contextualises service delivery in relation to socio-cultural and economic factors because gender neutral approaches fail to meet the "unique treatment needs of women" (Judd et al., 2009, p. 109).

Feminist Research and Ethics of Care

The ethical approach to research that is now common emerged out of a history of unethical research undertaken with little respect for participants' rights, dignity or wellbeing (for more see Jarldorn, 2014). Much has changed since then, with university human research ethics committees acknowledging that social sciences research creates human connections, and that those connections must be respectful. Our feminist practice of research is guided by a feminist research ethics of care, an approach developed since the second wave of feminism that continues to be nuanced by third and fourth-wave feminist researchers.

Ethical research "values the well-being of participants and researchers alike, working to actualise human flourishing not just through research outcomes but through the very practice of research itself" (Peake & Sharp, 2024, p.27). This is a very different take on research to traditional, masculinist positivist approaches. Taking this further, ethical research should centre the critical practice of care and "reciprocal, accountable relationships across difference" (Peake & Sharp, 2024, p.27). There is value in recognising our own limitations around ways of knowing to better understand intersectional structures of oppression but also to work towards dismantling them by highlighting the centrality of social context, relationships and power to the problems we study. This, in turn, rests on awareness of the affective and emotional impact of research on participants, including its potential harms, and the relationships formed in the research process (Peake & Sharp, 2024). In expanding a feminist ethics of care to a feminist *research* ethics of care, Miele et al. (2024) argue that "Western research 'norms' are associated with naturalistic or positivist approaches that typically guide participant recruitment, data collection methods and overall study design" (p. 126) while a feminist research ethics of care takes research "back into a gendered position of carer rather than researcher" (p. 138).

Undertaking Feminist Participatory Action Research

In the final section of this chapter, we outline the principles that guided our approach to feminist co-designed action research with young women; the concrete steps we took are outlined in later chapters. Jackson et al.'s (2024) recent editorial, *Positionality in Critical Feminist Scholarship*, provides a useful checklist of points for researchers to consider throughout the research process in order to reflect upon "questions of power, oppression, privilege, and social location as we design, conduct, and write up our research" (pp. 8–9). The editorial, while pitched at authors seeking to publish in the feminist social work journal, *Affilia*, provides a relevant framework for all feminist researchers to consider throughout their work from project development through to authorship. They write:

1. What is the researcher's relationship to the topic of this study, people, and communities of study? How is the researcher's social position and lived experience situated vis-à-vis the people and communities—and what are the relationships of power embedded within these relationships? How should these considerations of power be described in the manuscript?
2. Where and with whom was this research conducted? In what ways were researchers insiders and outsiders with regard to the populations and phenomena studied?
3. Who are the various collaborators/team members on the research project, and what are their relationships?
4. How were the research questions developed? Who was involved?
5. How will the research process and outcomes harm and/or benefit the people and communities in the study of focus? How can harms be mitigated and positive outcomes be enhanced—and how will the subjects of study be involved in these determinations?

6. Who funded or supported this research? How did that shape who participated, how the research was conducted, and how findings were disseminated?
7. How were data determined, sourced, and collected? Who participated in the data collection process?
8. How were data analysed? What frameworks and assumptions were used? Who participated in data analysis and interpretation?
9. How did the positionality of the researchers and participants influence the data collection and analysis process? What challenges and opportunities emerged?
10. How has historical, political, and social context been described and accounted for in both the research process and write-up?
11. What institutional barriers were encountered in this research process, and how were they navigated?
12. How did researchers with privilege and access to institutional power use it in ways to benefit the people and communities served by their research and also attend to their own personal and professional goals?
13. Where and how is a discussion of positionality and its influence on the process and substance of the research included in the manuscript? How does the placement of positionality within the article (e.g., at the beginning vs. at the end) support transparency and consideration of social location throughout an article (as opposed to an afterthought)?
14. What dialogue has taken place around authorship order?
15. Should this research be done or have been done in the first place based on the answers to these questions? If not, what opportunities for corrective actions and/or reparations exist? (Jackson et al., 2024, pp. 8–9)

Questions like these shaped the methodology used in this research project, right through from its early conceptualisation to working together on the outputs, including this book.

The Connections Between Co-Design, Action Research and Feminism

Typically, participatory action research involves creating spaces in which participants engage together in cycles of critical reflection and action. This is not just a tick-box exercise in inclusivity, though, but offers a vital contribution to the creation of new knowledge, as it seeks to make porous the walls between academia and the community. Generating theory and knowledge, is not limited to academia, but is a practice undertaken by all humans (Frisby et al., 2009, p. 15), even if they are not aware of it. However, participatory action research is best understood not as a methodology or a set of techniques, but as "an approach or orientation to inquiry" (Aziz et al., 2011, p. 306). Furthermore, participatory action research has a

> strong affiliation with feminism…namely the participatory nature of the process, its critical stance towards social power structures, its democratic worldview, and its commitment to achieving social change through a combination of generation of knowledge and action in 'real life'. (Krumer-Nevo, 2009, p. 280)

As such, feminist action research provides fertile ground for the creation of new knowledge (Maguire et al., 2004, p. xiv). Similarly, Feminist Participatory Action Research (FPAR) can be understood as "a tool, not a panacea, that involves a particular way of looking at the world and interacting with research participants to overcome the androcentrism that characterises other types of research" (Reid et al., 2006, p. 316). Moreover, as Shimei and Lavie-Ajayi (2021) argue, "every FPAR is embedded in the socioeconomic, political and cultural contexts within which it takes place" (p. 273).

Connecting These Ideas to Our Project

Considering the prevalence of sexual assault, family and domestic violence, it would be reasonable to expect that even in a relatively small research project like ours, it is likely that members of the research team will share at least some experiences of gendered oppression with participants, in both social and mental health contexts. Rather than viewing these collective experiences negatively, a shared understanding of them has the potential to generate nuanced research questions, and more empathetic approaches to data collection and analysis. We also believe that a team made up entirely of women enabled us to be better equipped to navigate ethical considerations, be attuned to intersectional issues, cultural sensitivities and the gender dynamics that influence women's experiences. We argue that taking this approach can lead to the creation of gender and culturally appropriate research methods and co-produced interventions. It was clear to us that our shared experiences and overlapping identity markers made building trust and rapport with our participants and each other feel natural, helped mitigate power imbalances, and led to open, honest and sensitive communication throughout our data collection and interactions with participants. As noted earlier, in later chapters, we explain in detail the concrete steps undertaken in the process of co-designing and undertaking our action research project with young women.

Limitations

Like any research methodology, the approach we used for our project does have its limitations. It is unlikely that we could replicate the outcomes of our project if we had set out to create a peer-to-peer resource for young men. Nor would we be the right team to undertake a project like this with Indigenous communities; no amount of learned cultural sensitivity can replace embodied lived experience or the right for Indigenous peoples to reclaim their voice through decolonising approaches to research (Tuhiwai Smith, 2012). A further limitation is that when co-designing resources that involve the development of technology-based interventions specifically for women, we found that the lack of women in STEM and tech-based roles became problematic. It took us many weeks to find a woman tech designer to work with us, and we are indebted to her for her feminist orientation to the project. While the number of women in these roles is growing, it remains low compared to the number of men, while those women who do exist in this profession are in high demand.

Conclusion

Finally, we should caution that taking a critical, feminist approach to research, teaching and understanding the world more broadly is not without risk. Challenging long-held views about women's 'place' in the world can engender the risk of violent responses (Gibson et al., 2024), reminding us that little has changed in the years since Park et al. (2017) lamented that "we do not live in a postgender world" (p.7). Even without threats of violence, overtly challenging through research medicalised explanations of female distress that overlook women's oppression rarely attract research funding or the provision of services outside of the psycho-medical paradigm. As Gibson et al. (2024) recently warned in relation to social work research but their point applies more broadly, "It is certainly a tough time to do critical feminist scholarship in social work, which is why such scholarship is so very necessary" (p. 197). This last sentiment reflects our commitment to undertake this project with young women in the context of rising reports of psychological distress but with a keen focus on their strengths and living experience knowledge. In the first half of this book, we have laid the groundwork for our project. In the chapters that follow, we move from exploring theory to enacting it, offering a detailed account of the methods, decisions, learnings and outcomes that brought this project to life.

References

Ackerly, B., & True, J. (2010). Back to the future: Feminist theory, activism, and doing feminist research in an age of globalization. *Women's Studies International Forum, 33*(5), 464–472. https://doi.org/10.1016/j.wsif.2010.06.004

Aziz, A., Shams, M., & Khan, K. S. (2011). Participatory action research as the approach for women's empowerment. *Action Research, 9*(3), 303–323. https://doi.org/10.1177/1476750310396952

Brown, B. (2024, March 5). Women still underrepresented in Australian parliaments. *The Australia Institute.* https://australiainstitute.org.au/post/women-still-underrepresented-in-australian-parliaments/

Crenshaw, K. (1991). Mapping the margins: Intersectionality, identity politics, and violence against women of color. *Stanford Law Review, 43*(6), 1241. https://doi.org/10.2307/1229039

Davis, G., & Khonach, T. (2020). The paradox of positionality: Avoiding, embracing, or resisting feminist accountability. *Fat Studies, 9*(2), 101–113. https://doi.org/10.1080/21604851.2019.1628604

Franzway, S. (2016). The sexual politics of citizenship and violence. *Women's Studies International Forum, 58*, 18–24. https://doi.org/10.1016/j.wsif.2016.04.006

Franzway, S., Moulding, N., Wendt, S., Zufferey, C., & Chung, D. (2019). *The sexual politics of gendered violence and women's citizenship.* Policy Press. https://doi.org/10.1332/policypress/9781447337782.001.0001

Frisby, W., Maguire, P. & Reid, C. (2009). The 'f' word has everything to do with it: How feminist theories informaction research. *Action Research, 7*(1), 13–29. https://doi.org/10.1177/1476750308099595

Gavey, N. (2005). *Just sex? The cultural scaffolding of rape.* Routledge.

Gibson, M. F., Diaz, M., & Karandikar, S. (2024). Critical feminism under critical conditions: Violence, silence, and resistance. *Affilia, 39*(2), 197–201. https://doi.org/10.1177/08861099241245167

Hamdani, Y., Kassee, C., Walker, M., Lunsky, Y., Gladstone, B., Sawyer, A., Ameis, S. H., Desarkar, P., Szatmari, P., & Lai, M.-C. (2023). Roadblocks and detours on pathways to a clinical diagnosis of autism for girls and women: A qualitative secondary analysis. *Women's Health, 19*. https://doi.org/10.1177/17455057231163761

Hanisch, C. (1970). The personal is political. In S. Firestone & A. Koedt (Eds.), *Notes from the second year: Women's liberation* (pp. 76–78). Major Writings of the Radical Feminists.

Jackson, K. F., Goodkind, S., Diaz, M., Karandikar, S., Beltrán, R., Kim, M. E., Zelnick, J. R., Gibson, M. F., Mountz, S., Miranda Samuels, G. E., & Harrell, S. (2024). Positionality in critical feminist scholarship: Situating social locations and power within knowledge production. *Affilia—Feminist Inquiry in Social Work, 39*(1), 5–11. https://doi.org/10.1177/08861099231219848

Jarldorn, M. (2014). The politics of research ethics in social work: Reflections from a first-time researcher. *Journal of Social Work Values and Ethics, 11*(2), 52–60.

Jenkins, K. (2021). *The gendered costs of childcare: A feminist analysis of the effects of Australia's early childhood education and care system on women's inequality in the workforce and beyond*. The University of Melbourne. https://www.unimelb.edu.au/__data/assets/pdf_file/0007/4117192/Kate-J_FoWL-Report.pdf

Judd, F., Armstrong, S., & Kulkarni, J. (2009). Gender-sensitive mental health care. *Australasian Psychiatry, 17*(2), 105–111. https://doi.org/10.1080/10398560802596108

Kim, M. E. (2018). From carceral feminism to transformative justice: Women-of-color feminism and alternatives to incarceration. *Journal of Ethnic & Cultural Diversity in Social Work, 27*(3), 219–233. https://doi.org/10.1080/15313204.2018.1474827

Kim, M. E. (2020). Anti-carceral feminism: The contradictions of progress and the possibilities of counter-hegemonic struggle. *Affilia, 35*(3), 309–326. https://doi.org/10.1177/0886109919878276

van der Kolk, B. A., Hostetler, A., Herron, N., & Fisler, R. E. (1994). Trauma and the development of borderline personality disorder. *Psychiatric Clinics of North America, 17*(4), 715–730.

Komaroff, A. L., & Lipkin, W. I. (2023). ME/CFS and long COVID share similar symptoms and biological abnormalities: Road map to the literature. *Frontiers in Medicine, 10*. https://doi.org/10.3389/fmed.2023.1187163

Krumer-Nevo, M. (2009). From voice to knowledge: Participatory action research, inclusive debate and feminism. *International Journal of Qualitative Studies in Education, 22*(3), 279–295. https://doi.org/10.1080/09518390902835462

Lambert-Patel, T. (2020, August 16). 'Why didn't she cry?' How Lindy Chamberlain became the poster child for life-shattering gender bias. *Women's*

Agenda. https://womensagenda.com.au/latest/why-didnt-she-cry-how-lindy-chamberlain-became-the-poster-child-for-life-shattering-gender-bias/

Lennane, K., & Lennane, R. (1973). Alleged psychogenic disorders in women–A possible manifestation of sexual prejudice. *The New England Journal of Medicine, 288*(6), 288–292. https://doi.org/10.1056/nejm197302082880605

Macdonald, F. (2024). Neoliberal care policies and women's economic inequality. In P. Toner & M. Rafferty (Eds.), *Captured: How neoliberalism transformed the Australian state* (pp. 175–194). Sydney University Press.

Mackay, F. (2015). *Radical feminism: Feminist activism in movement.* Palgrave Macmillan.

Mackay, F. (2021). Raising awareness and improving responses to gender-based violence: The contribution of feminist thought and activism. In C. Bradbury-Jones & L. Isham (Eds.), *Understanding gender-based violence: An essential textbook for nurses, healthcare professionals and social workers* (pp. 3–14). Springer. https://doi.org/10.1007/978-3-030-65006-3

Maclean, M., & Groves, D. (2024). *Women's issues in social policy.* Taylor & Francis.

Maguire, P., Brydon-Miller, M., & McIntyre, A. (2004). Introduction. In M. Brydon-Miller, P. Maguire, & A. McIntyre (Eds.), *Traveling companions: Feminism, teaching, and action research* (pp. ix–xviii). Praeger.

McNay, L. (2004). Agency and experience: Gender as a lived relation. *The Sociological Review, 52*(2_suppl), 175–190. https://doi.org/10.1111/j.1467-954x.2005.00530.x

Meyers-Pantele, S. A., Ma, J., Horvath, K. J., Yu, I., Logie, C. H., Rafful, C., & Earnshaw, V. A. (2024). Experiences of gender-based stigma in health care in North America: A mixed-methods scoping review and synthesis of the literature. *Women's Health Reports, 5*(1), 867–888. https://doi.org/10.1089/whr.2024.0084

Middleweek, B. (2017). Dingo media? The persistence of the "trial by media" frame in popular, media, and academic evaluations of the Azaria chamberlain case. *Feminist Media Studies, 17*(3), 392–411. https://doi.org/10.1080/14680777.2016.1235054

Miele, R., Root, J., Godderis, R., & Meerai, S. (2024). Towards a Feminist Research Ethics of Care: Reflections, Lessons, and Methodological Considerations for Doing Research During a Pandemic. *Studies in Social Justice,18*(1), 125–142.

Moulding, N. T. (2016). *Gendered violence, abuse and mental health in everyday lives: Beyond trauma.* Routledge. https://doi.org/10.4324/9781315816630

Moulding, N. (2019). 'We never quite measure up, do we?' An intersectional approach to mothering and mental health. In C. Zufferey & F. Buchanan (Eds.), *Intersections of mothering: Feminist accounts* (pp. 168–179). Routledge.

Mulvey, A., Terenzio, M., Hill, J., Bond, M. A., Huygens, I., Hamerton, H. R., & Cahill, S. (2000). Stories of relative privilege: Power and social change in feminist community psychology. *American Journal of Community Psychology, 28*(6), 883–911. https://doi.org/10.1023/a:1005120001986

Munch, S. (2004). Gender-biased diagnosing of women's medical complaints: Contributions of feminist thought, 1970–1995. *Women & Health, 40*(1), 101–121. https://doi.org/10.1300/j013v40n01_06

Oxfam, (n.d.). Why the majority of the world's poor are women. https://www.oxfam.org/en/why-majority-worlds-poor-are-women

Park, Y., Wahab, S., & Bhuyan, R. (2017). Feminism in these dangerous times. *Affilia, 32*(1), 5–9. https://doi.org/10.1177/0886109916686271

Peake, L., & Sharp, W. (2024). Feminist research ethics. In L. Peake, N. Razavi, & A. Smyth (Eds.), *Doing feminist urban research: Insights from the GenUrb project* (pp. 117–129). Routledge.

Reid, C., Tom, A., & Frisby, W. (2006). Finding the 'action' in feminist participatory action research. *Action Research, 4*(3), 313–330. https://doi.org/10.1177/1476750306066804

Risse, L. (2024, November 20). Women are still being paid almost $30,000 a year less than men and the gap widens with age. *The Conversation*. https://theconversation.com/women-are-still-being-paid-almost-30-000-a-year-less-than-men-and-the-gap-widens-with-age-243941

Shimei, N., & Lavie-Ajayi, M. (2021). Four practices for conducting feminist participatory action research with young women. *Action Research, 20*(3), 261–277. https://doi.org/10.1177/14767503211036489

Smith, D. (1987). *The everyday world as problematic: A feminist sociology*. University of Toronto Press.

Srivarathan, A. (2022). 'You are kind of like one of us': Exploring researcher positioning in studying community-based health promotion interventions among social housing residents of Danish, Turkish and Pakistani origin. *Qualitative Health Research, 32*(4), 599–608. https://doi.org/10.1177/10497323211067523

Stewart, S. (2021). A mother's love knows no bounds: Exploring 'good mother' expectations for mothers involved with children's services due to their partner violence. *Qualitative Social Work, 20*(3), 681–702. https://doi.org/10.1177/1473325020902249

Taylor, J. (2021). *Why women are blamed for everything: Exposing the culture of victim-blaming*. Constable.

Taylor, J. (2022). *Sexy but psycho: How the patriarchy uses women's trauma against them*. Constable.

Thompson, J., & Blake, D. (2021). Women's experiences of medical miss-diagnosis: How does gender matter in healthcare settings? *Women's Studies Journal, 34*(1), 22–36. https://doi.org/10.26686/wgtn.14198627

Tuhiwai Smith, L. (2012). *Decolonizing methodologies: Research and indigenous peoples*. Zed Books.

Weedon, C. (1996). *Feminist practice and poststructuralist theory* (2nd ed.). Wiley-Blackwell.

Westmore, B. (2024). *Fully realising the economic potential of women in Australia*. Organisation for Economic Co-operation and Development. https://www.oecd-ilibrary.org/docserver/3470e5d8-en.pdf?expires=1732390901&id=id&accname=guest&checksum=C7EFF32A41E3236A7062FC76B23B47C4

Zufferey, C., & Buchanan, F. (2019). Introduction: Theorising intersectional feminism and mothering. In C. Zufferey & F. Buchanan (Eds.), *Intersections of mothering: Feminist accounts* (pp. 1–12). Routledge. https://doi.org/10.4324/9780429430411

CHAPTER 5

Creating Safe Spaces to Explore Young Women's Experiences of Mental Health and Help-Seeking

Nicole Moulding, Michele Jarldorn, and Kate Deuter

Abstract This chapter tracks the development and rollout of our survey and online focus groups. We set out our research aims, describe the development of our online qualitative survey and how we used that to recruit participants for our online focus groups and co-design workshops. During the first focus group, the young women provided deeper context to the survey responses. This collective approach to the study provided the young women with a safe space to hear and share experiences, exercise choice and control, and enabled collaboration and relationship building. Such an approach is critical to co-designing new online mental health resources and supports tailored to the unique mental health needs and gendered experiences of young women.

Keywords Online qualitative survey • Co-design • Feminist theory • Young women • Mental health • Peer support

---

N. Moulding · M. Jarldorn (✉) · K. Deuter
University of South Australia, Magill, SA, Australia
e-mail: Nicole.Moulding@unisa.edu.au;
Michele.jarldorn@unisa.edu.au; Kate.Deuter@unisa.edu.au

M. Jarldorn et al. (eds.), *Feminist Action Research in Mental Health*, https://doi.org/10.1007/978-3-032-04406-8_5

Introduction

In the early chapters of this book, we explored the evidence attesting to young women's disproportionate experiences of poor mental health, the scope for peer-to-peer work in mental health and situated our thinking within a feminist framework. In this chapter, we begin by describing some of the project's practicalities before moving on to share what we learned from our qualitative survey and online focus groups with young women, where we sought to explore deeper explanations of the survey responses. The initial idea for this project stemmed from the discovery of the UK organisation *Agenda Alliance*, which provided online and in-person mental health support to young women from diverse backgrounds in ways that took into account the gendered social contexts in which they lived. The website and associated services linked to *Agenda Alliance* were shaped and informed by feminist thinking and took a political, activist and advocacy approach to the information and resources it provided. We wondered if something similar would help support young women in their mental well-being in an Australian context. Our project was funded by a local philanthropic body, the Breakthrough Mental Health Research Foundation, which was open to researchers who took a broader social view of mental health research and recognised the value of offering choices for users of mental health services.

The overarching aim of the project was to investigate the potential for gender-responsive mental health peer support for young women in Australia. Our aims over the two stages of funding were:

- To review the evidence on models of mental health peer support for young women.
- To investigate young women's experiences of services and preferred models of support.
- To co-design a peer-informed, gender-responsive mental health website and resources for young women.

As we explained in earlier chapters, our study adopted an action-oriented and participatory feminist research approach informed by an intersectional understanding of young women's oppression. Designed well, participatory and action-oriented research should be experienced as inclusive by participants (Jarldorn, 2022). Applying this inclusivity to a technology-based project like this requires the involvement of end-users throughout the project (co-design), where participants work in collaboration with the research team and a website creator, rather than only obtaining feedback on a finished product (consultation). However, we also acknowledge that community members have busy lives and that participating in a research project is unlikely to be their priority, no matter how important or relevant the topic is to their lived experience. Because of this, we sought to actively engage young women throughout the study by offering varying levels of participation, from responding to an anonymous survey, contributing to our online focus groups, right through to involvement in the online co-design workshops, speaking at the project knowledge exchange and co-authorship (see Chap. 7).

Designing the Online Survey

Online qualitative surveys have the potential to gather rich data, especially if they are well-designed and the distribution method is targeted and well-planned (Terry & Braun, 2017). After reviewing the evidence on young women's mental health and service gaps, we developed a survey tool to explore their experiences of mental health and wellbeing and their preferred modes of support, taking great care to word the questions clearly and inclusively. Through this process, we refined what we meant by 'young women', turning to the 18- to 30-year age range used by large research-based government-funded bodies such as the Australian Bureau of Statistics (ABS) and the Australian Institute of Health and Welfare (AIHW); the survey was open to all individuals in this age group who identified as women or as non-binary. We reviewed the wording used in other mental health surveys as a guide for asking questions about levels of education, income and location of residence. We began the survey by asking about caring responsibilities, mental health challenges and current mental health, relationship status and family history. We then moved to ask questions that sought to understand previous experiences of accessing mental health support. Before releasing the survey, we asked young women we knew—daughters, friends and colleagues—to pilot the survey questions to ensure we got the language and tone right, making revisions where necessary based on their feedback. After gaining ethics approval from the University of South Australia Human Research Ethics Committee (#203550), we released the survey, promoting participation via community organisations and our university's social media channels. The survey was available to complete online between June and September 2021 and was open nationally to anyone self-identifying as a woman or non-binary person aged 18–30 years old. Fifty-two young women completed the survey. We monitored the survey responses as they were submitted and made the decision to close the survey once we began receiving similar responses because responses had reached a sufficient level of data saturation. The decision to close the survey was driven by the idea of 'information power' (Malterud et al., 2016), which is determined by a combination of appropriate study aims, sample specificity, questions posed, and the analysis strategy deployed. We used qualitative content analysis to condense the extensive and varied raw text to explore and interpret the data and establish links between our research objectives and our interpretation of the data (Elo et al., 2014).

Our Sample

While the study did not seek a representative sample in the strict sense of the term, the 52 young women who completed the online survey were representative of the main groups of young women in the Australian population. The table in Fig. 5.1 shows the demographic diversity among participants was represented across age, sexuality, cultural histories, health, ability and location. Most of the young women were in lower-income groups. The sample also included significant representation from gender and sexually diverse young women, and a reasonable proportion of young women from culturally diverse backgrounds, although young Aboriginal women were under-represented. Most participants lived close to a capital city, all but two had completed high school, with 20 respondents indicating they had completed a bachelor's degree or higher. Most were earning well under the median weekly Australian wage.

Survey Findings

Analysis of the qualitative responses confirmed that young women largely understood their experiences of mental health challenges as connected to gendered violence and other forms of gendered social inequality and discrimination. For example, one participant wrote:

> My experiences with mental health and many of my friends' experiences with mental health issues have been sparked by men. Sexual assaults, rape and even general societal norms that make women feel as though they are

Characteristics	Category	Number
Gender identity	Woman she/her	48
	Non-binary	4
Sexuality	Hetero/straight	27
	Queer	12
	Bisexual	8
	Lesbian/Gay	3
	Prefer to self-describe	2
Age	18–22	19
	23–26	18
	27–30	15
Language/Culture	Aboriginal or Torres Strait Islander	1
	CALD	14
	Anglo	37
Disability/chronic health condition	No	44
	Yes	8
Location	Close to a capital city (metro area)	29
	Outer suburbs of a capital city	15
	In, or close to, a regional centre	5
	Rural area	3
Highest level of education	Year 10	1
	Year 11	1
	Year 12	18
	Advanced diploma	11
	Bachelor's degree or higher	21
Annual income AUD	Under 20k	16
	20k–30k	10
	30k–49k	13
	50k–69k	4
	70k–89k	4
	90k +	2
	Prefer not to say	3

Fig. 5.1 Demographics of our online survey participants (Moulding et al., 2024, p. 229)

> inferior are really the core reasons my friends have sought mental health support.

Another participant described multiple layers of violence they had experienced, saying:

> I witnessed human trafficking when I was overseas. I was around a lot of violence in my childhood and my aunt was murdered by her husband. Many

> female members of my family have experienced sexual abuse and rape, including myself….

Other participants said in reference to how they understand their mental health experiences:

> I was raped by an older school friend when I was 12.
>
> [M]y PTSD has been influenced by experiences of sexual harassment and abuse.

Many of the responses spoke to the ways that participants' gendered experiences had been minimised or entirely dismissed by mental health professionals. The question "what do you believe contributed to your mental health challenges?" led to responses that specifically point to service failures. For example:

> ignorant health professionals, [mental health] not being associated with particular types of experiences, [un]heard by doctors.

We also asked participants if they had ever drawn upon their own experiences to support others in their family or peer group, and alternatively, if they had ever been on the receiving end of such supports. They told us:

> I know that having someone listen non judgementally and holding space for someone else's big emotions is one of the best things you can do for others. I also will provide techniques or knowledge I have picked up over the years if people close to me want them/may benefit from them….
>
> I talk about relevant experiences, so they feel less alone or more hopeful or less ashamed/feel less like a failure. My mental illness has helped me to be more tolerant and less judgemental and also how much it helps to have people give genuine compliments and words of affirmation and reassure them of things like that my friends are attractive, loveable, smart and I care for them….

This use of self described by participants points to the value of drawing on lived experience when it comes to understanding and responding to the challenges associated with mental health and can be valuable resource in addition to more formal options. We also found that there was an appetite for mental health and wellbeing resources specifically designed by and for young women. Some of the reasons offered by survey participants as to why this was seen as valuable can be seen below:

> [it] would offer a strong and true perspective which other young women would appreciate.
>
> young women might think of ideas and issues that someone else might not be aware of or realise.
>
> young women are far more likely to know what other young women will like.
>
> [because it's developed by] people who understand the struggles themselves.
>
> because, how would a man be able to understand, let alone design a support service for women.
>
> so often, things aimed at young women completely miss the mark because they are made by someone who clearly has no understanding of what it is like to be a young woman.
>
> the experience of young women is completely unique and has many pressures that others may not understand.
>
> Often, I get put off by mental health supports because they are not women, survivor led. I would like to be able to speak to people who have had similar experiences.

Often, the responses demonstrated a strong understanding of, and respect for, diversity and were critical of mainstream, professional services. For example, one participant said:

> most therapy research and diagnostic criteria are based on men, so a non-man approach to support that understands and considers the specific problems women face, particularly those with intersecting identities, would be beneficial to me.

Overwhelmingly, the survey respondents indicated that they understood the intersectional nature of the experiences of young people identifying as women or non-binary people, saying:

> Some struggles are very unique to women and especially those from certain backgrounds...I'm straight and Caucasian but it would be good to have support for lesbian, bisexual and transgender women and also Aboriginal women so they can feel safe and supported by peers and get specific information that can help them best....

We also asked why they might use or suggest using online resources to their peers. The responses considered the costs, accessibility and confidential nature of this type of resource:

> mental health treatment is very expensive and often inaccessible.
>
> mental health support is expensive and I can't currently afford it, plus it's convenient being able to do [it] whenever or in my own home.
>
> resources I can access at my own leisure would mean that I can work it into my already existing routines and schedule.
>
> having information about how to manage mental health problems that is easy to access or easy to understand is great for people to use to understand why they may be experiencing certain feelings or why it may be affecting their lifestyle…information about services that understand young women's lives would be another amazing option as being a young woman can be hard especially with the social media in our generation therefore having more information that is specialised in that area would be beneficial.

There were many more responses like those above, demonstrating a significant appetite for online resources that consider young women's gendered experiences. Given that most participants indicated that they were earning well under the minimum wage in Australia (*at the time of writing, the minimum wage in Australia is around $49,000, see Fair Work Ombudsman, 2024), and the lengthy waiting times to see a mental health professional (Squires, 2023), access to resources that are free, and can be accessed immediately, would make a welcome addition to existing supports.

In addition to contributing valuable quantitative and qualitative data about the gendered nature of young women's mental health experiences, the survey responses overwhelmingly supported the idea of the usefulness of a peer-to-peer resource that would offer information curated by and for young women. A more detailed account of these survey findings is published elsewhere (see Moulding et al., 2024).

The Online Focus Groups

At the end of the survey, participants were invited to provide their contact details should they be interested in participating in an online focus group. Of the twenty-one respondents who initially left their contact details, eight young women joined us over two online focus groups.

Along with all having lived experience of mental health challenges, all focus group participants were either university graduates or current students in disciplines such as social work, speech pathology, psychology and similar allied health professions. The young women were from Adelaide, Melbourne and Sydney, with some already performing peer work in either a paid or voluntary roles. To prepare for the groups, we closely re-read the survey responses noting areas ripe for further exploration, and used these to iteratively create a framework of topics and questions to guide our semi-structured online focus groups. These included questions about the young women's understandings of peer support, whether they had used it, whether they would use it in the future and who they believed might benefit from it. We used ZOOM to hold the groups, which enabled young women from three states in Australia to participate. The groups were recorded, and later, transcribed verbatim, before we turned to analysing through content analysis what the young women told us.

The two online groups were co-facilitated by three members of the research team. The groups were lively with discussion and connection and ran for just over 90 minutes each. Rapport was built not just between the research team and the participants, but also between participants themselves. Through qualitative content analysis of the focus group transcripts, we identified four overarching themes: (1) 'Lived knowledge and shared power'; (2) 'Finding connection in a lonely place'; (3) 'The overwhelmingness of everything'; and (4) 'I'd use it...but...'.

'Lived Knowledge and Shared Power'

The young women's understandings of peer support were initially expressed in terms of its relationship to 'lived experience' shared experience and, even in the face of different experiences, shared feelings.

> [Peer support is] a good way to give support and a good service because it's definitely given by someone who knows what they're talking about from their own lived experience...not just an academic viewpoint of knowing the topic....
>
> Feeling validated by other young women....
>
> Even if you have a different experience [there is a] universality of emotions, of certain feelings....

As can be seen in these excerpts, there was some elevation of lived experience over professional knowledge along the lines that, 'the person knows what they are talking about...not just an academic viewpoint', with the second and third extracts emphasising the power of shared experience. The potential for professionals to share their own lived experiences with non-professionals was also raised in focus group discussions. This sharing of experience is an idea supported by Hewitt (2009, p. 373) who argues that lived experience perspectives have the potential to "create a climate for growth and change through the therapeutic use of self". Hence, shared lived experience was afforded great emphasis by the participants, including its potential to forge *'more equitable power relationships'*.

'Finding Connection in a Lonely Place'

Most of the young women who joined us in the online focus groups had not previously engaged in formal online mental health peer support, however, they had accessed a range of online mental health information and resources, including online forums and live chat functions. They told us that they had learned of these resources in diverse ways, including through mental health clinicians, university contacts, colleagues, friends and through the social media pages of community groups and established mental health providers. One of the participants indicated they had engaged in another study about online peer support and was more familiar with the process. Similar to observations from our survey data (Moulding et al., 2024), some of the young women expressed their preference for in-person, face-to-face conversations, but could also see the value in a unique online resource specifically designed for and by young women as an addition or alternative. This is supported by Muchamore et al.'s (2024) review of the literature on the provision of digital interventions that incorporate lived experience expertise, in that online interventions offer choice and convenience that can complement existing, traditional services. In terms of the specific perceived benefits of online support, most of the young women agreed it had the potential to alleviate feelings of isolation:

> I think for me, it really helps in terms of not feeling alone...which you know logically, you aren't. It's [when] you have that conversation with someone that's been in your shoes or a similar situation that you really feel that "oh, you get it!"....
>
> Not feeling alone, allowing myself permission [to not be okay]....

Not alone. Normalised by a normal-looking person....

For our participants, online support was also understood as normalising young women's problems. Turning to the group discussion about the barriers or challenges associated with online support, problems of accessibility and visibility were commonly mentioned, as well as issues with the online environment itself, such as having confidence in the reliability or accuracy of the information being provided:

> It's about being able to find them [the resources]....
>
> You know, like, Instagram influencers...a lot of them have their own wellbeing apps and wellbeing programs and you wouldn't know about that unless you were...and are they good?...
>
> [Especially]...when you're in the middle of an anxiety attack or just feeling like the world is falling apart and people aren't really saying anything, or it's taking a while to get a response, or the internet drops out...it can make you feel worse sometimes....

The comments presented above point to the need to ensure that online support can be easily located, is of high quality and is responsive to young women's needs at different points in time.

'The Overwhelmingness of Everything'

In exploring what might be distinctive about young women's needs for online mental health peer support, the focus group participants described the social contexts and contemporary issues they confronted in 'going out into the world'. Specifically, they talked about gendered violence; they expressed anxiety about climate change; the impact of COVID on young women; financial inequality and insecurity (and the concurrent need for more education in this area); fear of being unable to get into the housing market; workplace pressures; sexual health; birth control; raising children; disentangling the connection between their mental health struggles and their menstrual cycles; social media pressures (particularly surrounding body image and dieting culture) and the perception in society of young women as 'too sensitive' or 'too emotional'. These issues were also framed in terms of feeling invalidated:

> There needs to be more focused and catered support for women, especially in terms of... all of the day-to-day sexism that we experience, sexual harassment, assault. All of that.
>
> A lot of the time, we don't feel seen or heard....
>
> We all know that things have changed...but sometimes when you're in that therapeutic environment, it can quickly become a debate topic, rather than, umm...genuine concern....
>
> When you're younger and you're still learning...I think...the overwhelmingness of everything... can kind of become...a big thing. Even if it's just one tiny thing [like] 'I spilt my coffee on my pants today'. But it could be that whole day that joins onto that whole week. 'These are my last pair of pants; my washing machine broke, my power ran out and I can't afford my bill and I can't go to the laundromat'. It's nice to have someone [to talk to] that understands that it can happen all at once and can feel really overwhelming....

The young women pointed to the need for increased awareness of the specific needs of their generation, including acknowledgement and understanding of everyday sexism and assault and their impact, validation of their sense that society has rapidly changed rather than dismissal of their experiences and an understanding of the interconnectedness of problems in young women's daily lives.

'I'd Use it ... but ...'

The young women were open to the idea of engaging with an online mental health peer support website. However, the nature of website content was not their only concern. All of the young women agreed that they would use online peer support if it became readily available, even if (as most agreed) *'it didn't tick all the boxes'*.

> I think it's definitely about the information being shown to people, rather than people having to search for it ....
>
> I think if I grew enough of a trust, or like a bond, umm ... and if it is helpful and I do grow that trust ... I would pay for that sort of professionalism ....

Participants discussed some of the issues that would impact on their decisions to engage with an online resource; this included affordability, accessibility and developing trust in those running the resource. In our exploratory research at the start of this project, we also questioned the issue of affordability when exploring the potential for mental health Apps; we discuss this in the following chapter. Several young women also noted the need for supervision and moderation of such a site, and the importance of including links to in-person support at times when that might be more appropriate than obtaining support online.

Most of the young women in the focus groups pointed to the 'overwhelmingness' of many of the current mental health websites, 'with too many options' and 'not knowing where to go'. They discussed how some online website resources tried so hard to provide resources for every potential cohort, that it was hard to find information just for them. This led to a call for a minimalist look and feel, and that websites be 'very clear about what they offer':

> I personally find a lot of mental health websites really overwhelming...even the well-known ones. It's just like masses of information, so many different options, and I kind of just go...nope!

While they identified what an online resource should ***not*** look like, they were clear on the need for the site to be representative of the diversity:

> Definitely, with things like sexuality and disability. With sexuality, there's a lot of struggles that women go through in regards to that. Personally, I am part of that community. People questioning my gender identity, saying "well that doesn't make sense, you look like a girl"....

Although the young women expressed a specific desire for online resources that do not seek to cater for everybody, the importance of using an intersectional framework that catered to diversity was equally raised by participants, including consideration of respect for Aboriginal and Torres Strait Islander Peoples (the First Nations Peoples of Australia), class, sexuality and disability. The young women were adamant about the need for culturally inclusive language throughout. They also suggested the inclusion of short videos that would showcase a range of young women's lived experiences and online gaming as a potentially interesting and engaging tool that could be incorporated to increase interactivity.

Discussion

While the young women who participated in the survey and focus groups identified gendered violence and gender inequalities as significant contributors to their struggles around mental health, they also pointed more broadly to feeling overwhelmed by a wide range of anxieties in their daily lives, from housing and sexual health to body image issues and prejudice against young women. The most important omission from both face-to-face services and current online resources identified by the young women was the failure to acknowledge gendered violence and gender inequality as central to their struggles. More specifically, young women pointed to the role of gender inequality and violence in their poor mental health alongside experiences of a masculinist psycho-medical mental health system that omitted acknowledgement of these experiences. This finding justifies our theoretical perspective and its focus on understanding young women's mental health through a feminist lens that attends to both the material and symbolic gender inequalities in their lives and their impact on mental health and wellbeing.

In relation to online resources in particular, the young women told us that existing options were also often experienced as overwhelming. They indicated that, instead, they want a simple, easy-to-use website that can clearly articulate what is being offered to them specifically as young women. However, given that most of the participants in our survey indicated they were earning well under the average wage in Australia, it is understandable that their key recommendation was that online mental health resources be free to access. Participants also particularly emphasised the value of using lived experience in a meaningful way, especially in terms of advocacy in relation to young women's mental health.

The findings from our qualitative survey and our online focus groups point towards the ways that professionals can minimise the experiences of young women when they present with mental health concerns thereby overlooking what is likely to be a myriad of personal, interpersonal, sociocultural and structural difficulties. The young women's accounts of engaging with the mental health system indicate how "notions of 'mental illness' ultimately act as distractions from a number of broader social and political issues" which inform the "medical understanding of distress" (Tseris, 2016, p. 38). Feeling 'overwhelmed by everything' can therefore be better understood not as the individual failings of young women but as a normal response to gendered social inequality and the resulting challenges many young women face. These processes of dismissing the socio-political basis of many of the mental health problems faced by young women can be understood through the idea of the politics of ignorance, which refuses to know about the systemic and discursive gendered inequalities that frame and shape these experiences (Tuana, 2006). Tuana (2006) suggests that a politics of ignorance actively and consistently denies the unequal effects of male dominance and its effects on women; in the case of young women's mental health and its connections with gender inequality and gendered violence, this form of ignorance involves 'knowing that we do not know, but not caring to know', even though such knowledge exists and has been elaborated in young women's accounts of their personal experience as documented in research like ours and others.

Our findings confirm that viewing mental health peer support through a feminist, intersectional lens necessitates addressing the unique needs of young women, including their physical, sexual and psychological safety and security, and their diverse social identities—all critical to good mental health. However, these needs are too often systematically denied in healthcare and social service settings. One of the key things we learned in the focus groups was that current online resources provided by mental health support services work so hard at ensuring that they cover multiple diverse groups' needs that finding specific and relevant information for young women is difficult. We observed this ourselves as we audited available online mental health resources as part of our literature review (see Chap. 6 for more on this). Here, we saw that despite the overwhelming evidence connecting gender inequality and gendered violence with poor mental health for young women, there was minimal acknowledgement of this within the resources available. In contrast, the online focus groups provided young women with a safe space to share and hear experiences, exercise choice and control, and enabled the beginnings of a collaboration in a co-design process focused on developing online resources.

As we learned through our survey, focus groups and the existing evidence in this area, peer support models utilising a feminist, intersectional approach framing young women's distress in the context of their gendered lived experiences could be a welcome extension to in-person modes of supporting young women to navigate the mental health challenges they experience. As Muchamore et al. (2024) found there is a "strong consensus among those with lived experience on the potential of digital technologies to support mental health support, emphasising the importance of supplementing rather than replacing in-person support" (p. 4). More specifically, peer informed women's specific services can "provide spaces and support that recognise and address trauma in ways that are not undertaken in services that are male focused or are blind to the different needs and experiences of gender" (Andleeb et al., 2020, p.13).

At the end of this stage of the project, the young women reflected positively on their experiences. They were pleased that their decision to complete an online survey about their own mental health had led them to be involved in co-creating a solution that they could inform and shape. This idea is supported by a recent review on incorporating lived experience in digital mental health interventions, which recommends that people with lived experience should be engaged in authentic and meaningful ways (Muchamore et al., 2024). This study supports our choice to use an iterative approach to recruitment, data collection and analysis with the young women to develop and build their own online mental health intervention over time. Inclusive and participatory design that involves end-users and draws on co-design principles can have more social impact because it ensures that digital solutions fit with intended health outcomes and are the right approach for the intended audience (Antonini, 2021; Burkett, 2012). Our findings also point to the ways that young women with lived experiences of mental ill-health gain valuable support from sharing with others, including those from different demographic backgrounds with potentially different lived experiences, enabling new connections to be formed (see, e.g., Blanch et al., 2012). Our findings also indicate openness among young women to engaging in online support that specifically caters to their needs.

Based on our review of the existing evidence and our analysis of the survey and focus group data, as well as observations of the co-design process we commenced in this stage of the project, we make the following recommendations. First, existing mental health services could be more effective for young women if they incorporated gender-responsive, trauma-informed approaches that acknowledge the reality of gendered violence and other gender and social inequalities in young women's lives and their significant impact on mental wellbeing.

Second, there appears to be an appetite among young women themselves for online support as an adjunct to appropriate and effective in-person support. Within this, there is scope for the development of specialist sections devoted to particular sub-groups of young women, for example, Aboriginal young women, CALD young women, women who identify with diverse gender and sexual identities, and young women living with disability. Further research could evaluate the effectiveness and uptake of online peer support for diverse groups of young women that recognises histories of gendered violence as a likely contributor to their mental health challenges. Lastly, university programs that educate and train health professionals, including those in social work, nursing, medicine and psychology, need to include an understanding of the impact of gendered violence and other forms of gendered violence on young women's mental health with a focus on trauma-informed approaches in their curricula.

Conducting Research Online

We end our discussion with a reflection on using ZOOM to facilitate our online focus group data collection and analysis. Online video-conferencing applications like ZOOM offer both challenges and opportunities for researchers seeking meaningful data from focus groups (Falter et al., 2022). In our study, the young women were already familiar with online video-conferencing software and seemed unconcerned about irregular disruptions such as glitches in internet connections, which occasionally froze discussions mid-sentence. There were some important benefits to using the ZOOM platform that we would not have experienced in face-to-face focus groups. For example, women from three different states in Australia participated in the online focus groups, all doing so from their homes. For the research team, entering into the participants' homes, albeit virtually, we saw how the presence of some of their companion animals served as conversation icebreakers, facilitating the 'small talk' (Lambley, 2021) between the research team and participants in a way that facilitated the development of rapport. One of the other unanticipated benefits of using ZOOM for the online focus groups was the way it simplified the transcription process because the software ensured that only one person at a time could speak. Although this can slow robust discussions somewhat, 'live' focus groups can be difficult to transcribe as group members often will speak over each other, making it difficult for a transcriber to connect words spoken to a specific person. Using ZOOM provided the dual benefits of being protected by multiple layers of university IT protocols, was free for us to use and completed the transcriptions within minutes.

Conclusion

Our experience confirmed for us that bringing young women together to discuss mental health concerns in a safe and encouraging environment can be a positive experience for them. Their ideas for the creation of an online mental health resource by and for young women were innovative and inclusive of the diversity of young women's needs and experiences. When lived experience is used in ways that share power, with a focus on the 'we' rather than the 'me', it has the potential to promote social justice and equality for a group who do not have equitable access to support, or alternatively, who choose to avoid using formal mental health services. Connecting young women with others who are experiencing similar mental health challenges can provide a source of both comfort and validation of experience as they come to realise that they are not alone in their struggles. The sharing of strategies used by others who have been there before can be helpful in setting realistic expectations for themselves, expectations that are not embedded within a psycho-medical model which views mental ill-health as being a result of an individual's lack of capacity to function in a world that is unequal.

In the following chapter, we describe the website co-design process and outcomes in more detail, review online mental health interventions and describe how we worked with the young women in another round of online focus groups to learn about their design and functionality preferences to create a website wireframe. We also explore how gender can be taken into account in website design and outline how we collaborated with a website designer to bring the young women's ideas to life.

References

Andleeb, H., Parker, J., Mackay, T., Matthews, F., McWilliam, J., Haider, F., Iqbal, N., White, S., & Pinfold, V. (2020). *Evaluation of the women side by side project. Final report.* McPin Foundation and St George's University of London, UK.

Antonini, M. (2021). An overview of co-design: Advantages, challenges and perspectives of users' involvement in the design process. *Journal of Design Thinking, 2*(1), 45–60.

Blanch, A., Filson, B., Penney, D., & Cave, C. (2012). *Engaging women in trauma-informed peer support: A guidebook.* National Center for Trauma-Informed Care.

Burkett, I. (2012). An introduction to co-design. *Sydney: Knode, 12*, 12.

Elo, S., Kääriäinen, M., Kanste, O., Pölkki, T., Utriainen, K., & Kyngäs, H. (2014). Qualitative content analysis: A focus on trustworthiness. *SAGE Open, 4*(1). https://doi.org/10.1177/2158244014522633

Fair Work Ombudsman. (2024). *Minimum wages*. https://www.fairwork.gov.au/pay-and-wages/minimum-wages

Falter, M. M., Arenas, A. A., Maples, G. W., Smith, C. T., Lamb, L. J., Anderson, M. G., Uzzell, E. M., Jacobs, L. E., Cason, X. L., Griffis, T. A. N., Polzin, M., & Wafa, N. Z. (2022). Making room for Zoom in focus group methods: Opportunities and challenges for novice researchers (during and beyond COVID-19). *Forum, Qualitative Social Research, 23*(1). https://doi.org/10.17169/fqs-23.1.3768

Hewitt, J. (2009). Redressing the balance in mental health nursing education: Arguments for a values-based approach. *International Journal of Mental Health Nursing, 18*(5), 368–379. https://doi.org/10.1111/j.1447-0349.2009.00633.x

Jarldorn, M. (2022). Centering participants voices as inclusive research practice: Putting the voice into photovoice. In P. Liamputtong (Ed.), *Handbook of social inclusion: Research and practices in health and social sciences* (pp. 1351–1367). Springer. https://doi.org/10.1007/978-3-030-89594-5_72

Lambley, R. (2021). Small talk matters! Creating allyship in mental health research. *Qualitative Research in Psychology, 18*(4), 586–600. https://doi.org/10.1080/14780887.2020.1769239

Malterud, K., Siersma, V. D., & Guassora, A. D. (2016). Sample size in qualitative interview studies: Guided by information power. *Qualitative Health Research, 26*(13), 1753–1760.

Moulding, N., Jarldorn, M., & Deuter, K. (2024). What do young women want? Using a qualitative survey to explore the potential for feminist-informed mental health peer support. *Qualitative Social Work, 23*(2), 224–241. https://doi.org/10.1177/14733250221131598

Muchamore, I., Karanikolas, P., & Gooding, P. (2024). How lived experience expertise shapes research and development in digital mental health—A review of literature and insights. *SSRN Electronic Journal*. https://doi.org/10.2139/ssrn.4932039

Squires, M. (2023, January 14). Australia's suicide crisis: Mental health services overwhelmed. *The Advertiser*.

Terry, G., & Braun, V. (2017). Short but often sweet: The surprising potential of qualitative survey methods. In V. Braun, V. Clarke, & D. Gray (Eds.), *Collecting qualitative data: A practical guide to textual, media and virtual techniques* (pp. 15–45). Cambridge University Press.

Tseris, E. J. (2016). Thinking critically about 'mental health issues' affecting women during/after violence. *Social Alternatives, 35*(4), 37–42.

Tuana, N. (2006). The speculum of ignorance: The women's health movement and epistemologies of ignorance. *Hypatia, 21*(3), 1–19.

CHAPTER 6

Using Design Thinking and Bringing Ideas to Life

Michele Jarldorn, Jane Andrew, Kirstie Wyatt, Nicole Moulding, and Kate Deuter

Abstract This chapter begins by exploring the value of design thinking in creating mental health interventions. Drawing on a critical review of existing online health products and apps—as well as academic literature reviewed in earlier chapters—we detail how this material has informed our work. In the second half of the chapter, we reflect on the practical experience of developing the prototype in partnership with five young women in collaboration with the project's website designer. We also examine gendered preferences for digital design, young users' experiences with digital

M. Jarldorn (✉) · N. Moulding · K. Deuter
University of South Australia, Magill, SA, Australia
e-mail: Michele.jarldorn@unisa.edu.au; Nicole.Moulding@unisa.edu.au; Kate.Deuter@unisa.edu.au

J. Andrew
Coolbus Creative, Westbourne Park, SA, Australia
e-mail: jane@coolbuscreative.com.au

K. Wyatt
Wyatt Creative, Aberfoyle Park, SA, Australia
e-mail: kirstie@wyattcreative.com.au

M. Jarldorn et al. (eds.), *Feminist Action Research in Mental Health*, https://doi.org/10.1007/978-3-032-04406-8_6

mental health interventions, and how user experience (UX) and mental well-being intersect in this unique context.

Keywords Design thinking • Online health interventions • Online co-design workshops • Website

Design Thinking to Make a Difference

We deployed a design thinking methodology to take what we learned from our survey and focus groups to inform the creation of an online resource for young women. Design thinking consists of much more than making a product or service visually appealing. Instead, design thinking is "both a mindset and a set of practices that are solution based" …and is a… "fundamentally subjective practice that focuses on discovering the emotional needs of users, their idiosyncratic contexts, their motivational concerns, and other related entities" (Scholten & Granic, 2019, p. 4). Design thinking as a methodology requires interdisciplinary ideation, while its human-centred approach to developing programs and resources, where experimentation is participatory and 'empathy-driven' (Scholten & Granic, 2019; van der Westhuizen et al., 2020), aligns well with our own values as researchers and design practitioners. The combination of co-design and design-thinking extends the potential and scope of feminist research methods, with evidence suggesting that deploying design thinking and collaborating with potential end-users is a best practice approach to developing online mental health resources (Muchamore et al., 2024).

Putting Ideas into Action

While technology has significant potential to contribute to social good, we are also mindful of the harm technology mediated interventions can create and perpetuate (Bucic & O'Connor, 2024). We have incorporated this position into our feminist research ethics of care as we critically explore tech made *for* women across this chapter. This is because technology design reproduces the values held by its creators (D'ignazio & Klein, 2020), hence our purposeful recruitment of feminist women as research team members. This position also meets the feminist research ethics edict of 'do no harm' (Reid et al., 2011). As researchers, we are inspired by the work of the feminist collective Laboria Cuboniks (2018), who argue that

> technoscientific innovation must be linked to a collective theoretical and political thinking in which women, queers, and the gender non-conforming play an unparalleled role, and as feminists we should explicitly organise our feminist energies to repurpose technologies to re-engineer the world. (p. 17)

Although no single project alone could 're-engineer the world', we wanted this project to contribute to the availability of choices for young women. We believe that leveraging the potential of web-based interventions using a feminist framework offers a broader range of choices for young women seeking support for their mental health that are meaningful, authentic accessible and free.

A Feminist Critique of Online Health and Wellbeing Technologies

The last few decades have seen a boom in technology-based health interventions such as online resources, Apps and, more recently, artificial intelligence that are used to extend the support provided by health professionals, thus enabling more people to access health care on their own terms (Lau et al., 2025). Current market and industry trends for online platforms have been enabled and accelerated by the increased penetration of smartphones, and the expanding wireless network coverage. These technological advances provide digital health systems with new possibilities to address challenges associated with accessibility and timely support while offering more choices and reduced costs to service providers. However, while these various online supports and interventions have the potential to be helpful, technology-based interventions must be viewed critically, given that technology is shaped by the principles of power and wealth generation and steeped in the values of the coders and builders who create them (Madianou, 2021).

In one example of a critique of health technologies designed for women, Kissling (2006) revealed how negative portrayals of menstruation as a 'hygiene crisis' have been exploited to generate corporate profits, especially by 'femcare' industries. Technology has been used to extend this reach through the rapid development of Femtech. A combination of feminine and technologies (Balfour, 2023), Femtech refers to software and services designed specifically for women's health. Although Femtech addresses various aspects of women's health, its primary focus is on menstruation care through period-tracking apps. Such technology-based interventions in women's health use "gamification to elicit additional user data" while leveraging a "feminist rhetoric of empowerment" (Mathiason, 2023, p. 119). However, in reality, they use the neoliberal logics which expect 'good women' to be responsible for managing their health through "actionable health information" without consideration of social context (Mathiason, 2023, p. 128; O'Connor et al., 2025). This use of technology goes well beyond an information website like ours, but it is important to note that health and tech have become marketised (Mathiason, 2023), with women the consumer group spending the most on health-technology; however, the main beneficiaries of Femtech are biomedical corporations, not the women who use them (McMillan, 2022). Despite the focus on women's health, investment in women's health technologies "remains skewed away from products designed by and for women" (Balfour, 2023, p. 3).

The more recent rise of interventions using artificial intelligence, such as companion chatbots that have a specific focus on mental health and wellbeing, should also raise concerns; these include Woebot, a chatbot utilising cognitive behavioural therapy (CBT) principles primarily to older teens and young adults, offer text-based, personalised responses to user input. Woebot functioned by identifying potentially negative thoughts and offering options for better coping skills (Fitzpatrick et al., 2017). While the research by Fitzpatrick et al. (2017) found that these AI interventions were broadly useful, a recent study conducted by Eltahawy et al. (2024) was unable to replicate Fitzpatrick and colleagues' findings, while it was recently announced that Woebot chatbot will be decommissioned in mid-2025 due to ongoing ethical issues around online safety.

Another example of an AI 'companion' designed to improve mental wellbeing is Replika, marketed as "the AI companion who cares", using large language model (LLM) technology to evolve based on the 'conversations' it has with the user to become a companion. Replika claims to address loneliness, which is associated with poor mental health (see Courts et al., 2024). A study by Depounti et al. (2023) that focused on online discussion groups about using the paid, pro version of Replika that enables romantic relationships, found that the AI companion deployed "gendered imaginaries" of the ideal girlfriend, reproducing "rather stale narratives of gender and technology" (Depounti et al., 2023, p. 730). Some Replika users report being provided inappropriate or dangerous mental health advice, while the company owning Replika has been fined for breaching data privacy rules and not having any age verification systems in place (Reuters, 2025). Other critiques are that AI companions exploit human vulnerability, can be addictive, encourage violence towards others and expose minors to hypersexualised content. For a more detailed discussion on the pros and cons of mental health chatbots, see Snoswell et al. (2025) and Khawaja and Bèlisle-Pipon (2024).

Reviewing Existing Online Mental Health Apps for Young Women

The discovery phase of the design thinking process for this project commenced with a review of the literature, and the outcomes of our online survey and focus group research discussed in the previous chapter. Alongside this work, we reviewed some of the existing mental health Apps pitched at young women. We employed an international student studying for a Masters of Design, Pooja Kagraga to do this work. While no one individual experience can be considered representative of an entire cohort, as a young woman who uses multiple Apps, Pooja's online habits—for example, how she searches for and engages with online resources—provided us with useful insights into how young women might interact with these interventions.

Pooja reviewed thirty existing mental health and wellbeing Apps, using keywords to guide her search based on the qualitative responses from our online survey. There was a specific focus on the responses made to the questions around the following: (1) access to, the usefulness of, and enablers and barriers to online mental health information, and (2) the types of information and/or resources they would like to see available for young women online. The approaches applied fell across a spectrum from those targeting risk and protective factors in healthy individuals to those targeting individuals with a significant and or diagnosed mental illness (Donovan et al., 2022). The search found that mental health and wellbeing platforms primarily focus on the objectives of; (1) education and awareness; (2) diagnostic and treatment support; (3) disease and epidemic outbreak tracking, and (4) telehealth and telemedicine. Sitting beneath these objectives, the most common interventions identified included Cognitive Behavioural Therapy, Acceptance and Commitment Therapy, and Dialectical Behaviour Therapy, each of which sought to address mental health challenges ranging from stress, low self-esteem, poor sleeping habits and addictions. Some Apps had a focus on people who experience panic attacks, body image dysmorphia, grief, eating disorders or domestic violence, through to those diagnosed with anxiety, bipolar, depression, and borderline personality disorder. Common to all approaches in the Apps we reviewed was the focus on mental health literacy, improving people's knowledge about mental health and how mental wellbeing is fostered.

It should be noted that formal mental health diagnoses as described in the Diagnostic and Statistical Manual of Mental Illnesses (otherwise known as the DSM-5-TR) are contested (see, e.g., Davies, 2021; Taylor, 2023), and that we did not observe any Apps that acknowledged this alternative perspective, nor did they take a critical view of mental health and wellbeing. Given the increasing critiques of an emphasis on individualised, neoliberal responsibility for self-care and wellbeing (Kökçinar, 2022; Newcomb, 2021; O'Connor et al., 2025; Stuart, 2021), we believe this is a significant omission from the online resources we reviewed. We also note that none of the Apps reviewed indicated that they had been developed through engagement with the user experience. Although this may have occurred, the information was not prominent. It is therefore assumed that the App's design and content were created by 'experts in the field'.

Adoption, Engagement and Attrition

Despite their proliferation and potential effectiveness in supporting wellbeing, many evaluations of online mental health interventions have noted that they generally have high attrition rates (Orlowski et al., 2015; Alqahtani & Orji, 2020; Eltahawy et al., 2024). There are two key reasons for this. The first is based upon the mechanics and functionality of the App and often amounts to poor interface design and the content lacking specific information (Rapp & Cena, 2016). The second includes poor understanding of the target demographics. Lewis et al. (2020) suggest that gender and age play a specific role in attrition rates and that, most often, this is linked to the online intervention taking a generic approach to the user experience, which fails to target the intervention to specific gender and age cohorts. Although personalised Apps that take into account age, gender and other demographics are growing, little consideration has been paid to the potential for increases in digital inequalities (Bol et al., 2018). Bol and colleagues suggest there are realistic concerns around equity and access regarding paid Apps and, more importantly, risks to online privacy (Bol et al., 2018, p. 184).

More work is required by tech-based health information developers to define and understand the complexities of user engagement (Kaveladze et al., 2022). While interventions solely designed by industry are likely to have the most uptake—due to large and flexible funding models supported by assertive marketing techniques—interventions developed by academics are more likely to be based upon peer-reviewed and evidence-based interventions (Kaveladze et al., 2022). However, lived experience expertise contributions to the development of online Apps do not appear to have been considered to date.

Deciding to Create a Website

Our review of the academic literature on online mental health interventions, and of the Apps themselves, confirmed that creating a website rather than an App or chatbot was an appropriate strategy. We were clear that the online resource needed to be co-designed with young women to provide peer-informed and recommended knowledge and resources. Additionally, four key benefits of creating a website over developing an App became apparent early in the project design.

Time: Apps and other online tools require high-level tech skills and extensive testing for functionality and to find and remove 'glitches', whereas WordPress websites (as we used) work on a platform of tested functionality, widgets, and tools. This ensured that creating a website was achievable within the timeframe of our project.

Cost: The estimated cost of App building ranges from anywhere between $3000 and $250,000 (Gartner, 2024). None of these cost estimates factor in the App developer working in close collaboration with end users.

Ease of use: The back end of WordPress holds several similarities to the online learning systems used in our university and meant that a research team member could be taught to perform updates to the website once published. WordPress enabled us to create an open-access resource free from advertising.

eSafety: As we discussed earlier, young women's experiences of mental ill-health and gendered violence are connected to economic and financial abuse, which includes economic control (Postmus et al., 2020). Our review found that most online mental health interventions are based on a user-pays model, where often, a 'lite' version is accessible for free, but the full experience requires signing up for a monthly payment system—frequently connected to a credit card. Therefore, access and choice are conditional on the ability of the consumer to pay and have access to a credit card, and comes with the risks associated with using a credit card and the increasing incidence of auto-renewals. The risks around the collection of users' personal data, especially for women are high (Figueroa et al., 2021). It can also be difficult and frustrating to cancel an online subscription (Kemp, 2024; CPRC, 2024) and given the high attrition rates (Alqahtani & Orji, 2020, p. 2043) described earlier, actively avoiding adding another layer of distress to young women was an important consideration.

The Politics of Co-Design, Participation and Lived/Living Experience

While once a devalued position within the medical model of mental health (Foucault, 1967), people with lived and living experience of mental ill-health are increasingly recognised as invaluable contributors to understanding how "emotional distress is understood and managed in everyday life worlds" (Bennett, 2023, p. 49). Design guidelines for mental health technologies have to date mainly focused on systems that bring individuals with mental illness in contact with their service/support providers rather than peers (Andalibi & Flood, 2021). In a recent systematic review of the involvement of people with lived experience in the design and development of digital mental health technologies, Muchamore et al. (2024, p. 4) argue:

> Authentic and meaningful involvement of people with lived experience is essential for the further development of effective and ethical digital mental health technologies. Integrating their perspectives and expertise throughout the research process is crucial for addressing the diverse mental health needs of populations worldwide.

However, as we have indicated in earlier chapters, an acceptance of the quality and rigour of lived experience knowledge is not universal. As such, we find it useful to understanding participation in designing, developing and delivering health interventions as a political act. As Palmer et al. (2019) explain:

> Participation has become a distinct cultural and political movement characterised by user involvement in healthcare across a continuum encompassing

> shared decision-making in clinical treatments and management, quality improvement, service redesign and evaluation. This movement has seen a proliferation of approaches in healthcare quality improvement that use coproduction and related (though distinct) models of codesign, co-innovation and cocreation (p. 247).

Yet, the idea of co-design has been depoliticised, co-opted out of its more radical roots to become a mainstream approach with little weight placed upon the potential for the social good that co-design can offer (Jarldorn & Emery, 2024). One of the benefits of using co-design is that meaningful participation of community members and collaboration between scholar-activists can support "therapeutic activism" (Bryant et al., 2024, p. 8). While this activist approach to research may be uncommon, as we explained in Chap. 4, feminist research, by definition, challenges the status quo in its commitment to equality and social justice. Especially for feminist researchers located in social work, the idea of therapeutic activism is an approach that aligns with our goal of social justice, embedded in our codes of ethics (AASW, 2020). While Mullan (2023) argues that mental health therapy is a political practice, we propose that feminist research in mental health can similarly be political while continuing to offer mental and emotional healing.

The Online Co-Design Workshops

Five young women participated in the online co-design workshops. Three were current university students, while two were graduates who both indicated that they had some experience as peer workers; all were passionate about the idea of peer support for young women.. During the online workshops, the online design tool, 'Miro', provided a collaborative online platform for the young women to contribute to creating a virtual whiteboard. In preparation for the first workshop, participants were sent a link to our project Miro site and encouraged to familiarise themselves with the platform. During the first workshop, participants were oriented to the potential features of a website. We used a familiarisation activity by having participants using Miro to create and move post-it notes and insert text and images. This activity fostered discussion about existing online mental health support platforms, while Pooja shared with the young women what she had learned from her review of mental health Apps and websites. During the second half of the first session, we used the design thinking technique called 'Rose, Thorn and Bud'. This technique provides a feedback framework for participants to comment on what is positive or is already working, i.e., 'Rose', what is negative or not working, 'Thorn', while 'Bud' indicates areas of opportunity for a specific problem or topic (Datar & Bowler, 2015, p. 132). The young women provided feedback and ideas in relation to each of the three categories.

In the second workshop, participants were invited to distil the priorities they identified in the first workshop by rating from 1 to 5 those elements they felt were critical for a website. The next activity centred on identifying what they felt was an 'engaging' design for straightforward navigation. Based on a selection of four existing online mental health websites, participants were engaged in a conversation about the elements of the sites that they preferred or disliked. During the final activity, participants were invited to 'consider all things representative of the look and feel of a [successful] online mental health portal'. Participants were presented with images of various colours, shapes, and themes and invited to make selections from these images to create their personalised mood board.

During this session, and in common with the focus group feedback in the previous chapter, one of the most poignant things we learned was that most of the young women pointed to the 'overwhelmingness' of many of the current mental health websites, 'with too many options', and 'not knowing where to go'. They called for a more minimalist look and feel and noted the importance of websites 'being very clear about what they offer'. The importance of diversity was equally raised, including consideration of sexuality, culturally inclusive language and disability. As one of the final activities for Stage 1 of this project, we created a wireframe (or a bare shell) of a website, incorporating the suggestions provided by the young women. The prototype drew on the suggestions made by participants about strategies they used to maintain their wellbeing. We used images representing the diversity of young women and ensured that the wireframe was uncrowded with text and was easy to navigate.

We then met with co-design workshop participants and took them through the wireframe. From their feedback, we learned they wanted even more diversity in the images used, which were not airbrushed, as is typical of stock and open-access images commonly used in website construction. During the discussion, one of the participants suggested creating a photo submission portal on the website, where, once moderated and with appropriate permissions in place, they could be used on the website to represent diversity in respectful ways. This ability for young women to contribute to the website content was incorporated into the website design brief. The completed wireframe showed what the finished website might look like, but without the full functionality we dreamed of. The completion of the wireframe marked the completion of Stage 1 of the project. We explained to our participants that we were seeking funding for Stage 2 and were transparent in explaining that this funding was not guaranteed. Despite this, five of the young women expressed interest in participating in Stage 2.

The participants reflected positively on their experiences as participants and co-designers in Stage 1 and were pleased that their decision to complete an online survey about their mental health had led them to be involved in creating a solution that they could see, inform and shape. They spoke of their sense of achievement in seeing the website wireframe they had designed together, with one participant reflecting:

> It's been really cool, yeah, how we've done the survey, now this website, trying to figure out what we wanted, what you wanted, and now to be able to see a draft of it, yeah, I definitely wanna see how it continues.

Another woman spoke of the sense of comfort gained by the familiarity that had grown between participants across the co-design sessions, saying:

> I like the idea I suppose of seeing something come to fruition. It's nice to be able to see familiar faces as well.

Actively engaging with the young women across Stage 1 of the project was a meaningful experience for us. It provided a window into the context of young women's lives concerning their mental health, while their interactions with each other demonstrated the value of peer-to-peer support.

Collaborating with a Website Designer: Bringing Ideas to Life

We chose WordPress to host our project website because of its functionality, performance capacity and security, each of which was important for us. While applications like WordPress have enabled people to create their own websites without the need for long-term training or significant financial outlay, this increased accessibility does not always correlate with sophisticated content or seamless user experience. Our search of academic literature on gender and website design mostly resulted in publications that focussed on website design and user experience with regards to sales and marketing, rather than for health information. For example, a study by Djamasbi et al. (2007) found that gender plays a role in the preferred type and content used in websites, and a specific preference for the inclusion of images of people. The authors argued that "men and women respond more favourably to products designed by the member of their own gender, who tend to show different preferences in terms of images and colors when designing a website" (Djamasbi et al., 2007, p. 2). Later, Tsichla et al.'s (2016) exploration of gender preferences for website atmospherics noted that gender plays a role in perceptions, use patterns, purchase intentions, information search, satisfaction, online privacy and perceptions of risk.

There has been a growing body of research exploring the co-design of online mental health resources, particularly those involving young people as end users. Studies from Villatte et al. (2023), Calear et al. (2024), and Ludlow et al. (2023) each highlight the importance of creating digital platforms that are accessible, trustworthy, and responsive to the lived experiences and preferences of young users. Common recommendations from these studies include using calming and consistent visual designs, reducing text density, and incorporating interactive, personalised, and problem-solving content. Participants valued clear navigation, inclusivity, and features such as lived-experience stories, service cost and wait time transparency, and information tailored to diverse needs. Across these studies, co-design was shown to enhance user engagement and relevance, reinforcing the role of such digital tools as valuable complements to—not replacements for—face-to-face mental health support. These tools offer significant potential to improve access, particularly in rural and remote areas where services are often limited (Morgan et al., 2021; Kavanagh et al., 2023).

Designing for the User Experience

The User Experience—most commonly referred to as UX—refers to the overall experience a person has when interacting with a product, especially in digital contexts like websites. UX aims to incorporate every aspect of the way people interact with technology, taking into account their perceptions, emotions, preferences, and behaviours before, during, and after using the product. When UX design is done well, interactions with tech should be seamless, intuitive, efficient, and enjoyable for users (Aufderhaar et al., 2019). However, as Aufderhaar et al. (2019) point out, "the user experience is a complex and very subjectively perceived product characteristic" (p. 63). Yet much of the literature we reviewed on gender and UX is framed around simplistic, binaried and generalised notions of gender that are unhelpful, and point to the importance of using a feminist approach to website design.

When seeking to deploy feminist design principles in website design (see Feminist Principles of the Internet, n.d.), the following considerations around stakeholders, purpose and context are a useful guide:

1. "Rather than design for a 'universal user', can you identify a stakeholder who is not currently well served, and who could benefit from your design?
2. What might be some of the specific needs, barriers and problems that they face?
3. What are their strengths and viewpoints?
4. What different participatory methods do you have available so that your stakeholder can co-create or have direct input into the development of your design? Some examples of participatory methods include:
   - having a stakeholder from the community that you are designing for on your design team
   - ensuring community members agree you are addressing a relevant problem
   - ensuring that community members agree the choice of technology suits the solution they are seeking co-creation design workshops, early and ongoing feedback and testing". (Feminist Internet & Josie Young, n.d.)

When we began looking to employ a web designer for the project, our main criteria were that they needed to be open to working with a group of young women and be sensitive to their experiences. They needed to be open to this being an educative process of shared learning for everyone involved, rather than just a paid gig. This is how we met Kirstie.

Designing and Building Our Website

Kirstie worked with us on the project for around a year. We met online every two months with the five young women who chose to participate in the website design and build phase of the project. We set up a Trello site which the young women and the research team used as a repository for information, resources and ideas for the website. In between meetings, Kirstie would perform updates ready for the next session. During the website design sessions, Kirstie would share her screen so we could see what she was doing. We would pause to ask questions and work through various suggestions. Although this took longer than it would have if Kirstie just went away and constructed the site herself, the time spent was valuable, as we all learned what happens behind the scenes of the public face of a website.

Vu et al. (2021), p. 1325) explain there are five key design elements to consider when creating a website: information, navigation, graphics, information architecture and user interface. These design elements can only be achieved through completing four overlapping phases of discovery, design exploration, design refinement and finally the production phase. While some aspects of the initial prototype remain in the finished product, the completed version is far more sophisticated. Importantly, the five young women who worked on the website build with us have a strong sense of achievement and ownership of the final version because of their involvement in the decision-making along the way. Surprisingly, and counter to our approach, Vu et al. (2021) suggest that while "end-user input is important" when designing a website, "end users should not be allowed to direct the design process because the features they desire for the website may be hard to implement or may lead to a less than optimal design when all factors are considered" (p. 1326). Instead, the authors propose various 'hands-off' approaches to consultation and user testing. This advice is not only at odds with the principles of co-design; it also demonstrates how women's needs are rarely considered and understood when it comes to designing technology for women.

Reflections from Kirstie

One of the aspects I value most in design is the collaboration between designer and client, which is why co-design has always been central to my process. While I regularly consult with clients in my freelance work—discussing their needs, audience, and desired outcomes—the *peer2me* website project was my first experience working within a formal co-design team. This process expanded on my usual methods, involving the team deeply in every decision, from content and functionality to colours and images. Unlike typical client projects where visual choices are guided by communication goals and aesthetics, this collaboration prioritised how each design element made the young women feel. Their input shaped everything, including the website's name and imagery, which had to reflect authenticity and avoid the overly polished look common in mainstream mental health resources. This project reaffirmed that co-design can go beyond consultation—it can be a genuinely shared creative process.

The young women were very good at recognising clichès concerning gender and wellbeing. This was especially the case where the website wireframe had included an image of a lotus flower. As the women pointed out, images of lotus flowers are everywhere where women and wellbeing are advertised, often with yoga, meditation and even massage parlours! Once the research team heard this, we could not stop seeing lotus flowers in such settings—this is another example of how co-design offers such an enriching approach to the creation of services and interventions. I know that this experience has made me even more meticulous when choosing images, and I will carry this forward into future projects. Working with the research team and the young women in the co-design team was a rich and rewarding experience and made me realise just how inadequately women's needs are being met in the mental health space, and how much a resource like the website we have created was needed.

Conclusion

As we have described throughout this book, co-design requires the time to build and nurture working relationships that are far more complex than traditional applied research. We recommend that when co-designing technology-based interventions, great importance should be placed upon having the right people work with co-design participants. In the following chapter, we are joined by four of the five young women who worked with us to create the *peer2me* website as co-authors to reflect on their participation in project.

References

AASW. (2020). *Australian association of social workers code of ethics*. https://aasw-prod.s3.ap-southeast-2.amazonaws.com/wp-content/uploads/2023/08/AASW-Code-of-Ethics-2020.pdf

Alqahtani, F., & Orji, R. (2020). Insights from user reviews to improve mental health apps. *Health Informatics Journal, 26*(3), 2042–2066. https://doi.org/10.1177/1460458219896492

Andalibi, N., & Flood, M. (2021). Considerations in designing digital peer support for mental health: Interview study among users of a digital support system (buddy project). *JMIR Mental Health, 8*(1), e21819. https://doi.org/10.2196/21819

Aufderhaar, K., Schrepp, M., & Thomaschewski, J. (2019). Do women and men perceive user experience differently? *International Journal of Interactive Multimedia and Artificial Intelligence, 5*(6), 63–67. https://doi.org/10.9781/ijimai.2019.03.005

Balfour, L. (2023). Introduction: Who is FemTech for? In L. A. Balfour (Ed.), *FemTech* (pp. 1–19). Palgrave Macmillan. https://doi.org/10.1007/978-981-99-5605-0_1

Bennett, J. (2023). Visual communication and mental health. *Visual Communication, 22*(1), 46–70. https://doi.org/10.1177/14703572221130451

Bol, N., Helberger, N., & Weert, J. C. M. (2018). Differences in mobile health app use: A source of new digital inequalities? *The Information Society, 34*(3), 183–193. https://doi.org/10.1080/01972243.2018.1438550

Bryant, L., McFarland, B., & Andrew, J. (2024). Co-design communities of practice in community-based mental health and rural suicide prevention. *Design for Health, 8*(1), 4–24. https://doi.org/10.1080/24735132.2024.2317966

Bucic, T., & O'Connor, G. C. (2024). Avoiding harm in technology innovation. *MIT Sloan Management Review, 66*(1), 76–81.

Calear, A. L., Batterham, P. J., McCallum, S. M., Banfield, M., Moore, E., Johnson, N., & Morse, A. R. (2024). Designing a web-based navigation tool to support access to youth mental health services: Qualitative study. *JMIR Formative Research, 8*, e48945.

CPRC. (2024, August). *Let me out—Subscription trap practices in Australia*. Consumer Policy Research Centre. https://cprc.org.au/wp-content/uploads/2024/08/CPRC_LetMeOut_SubsTraps_Report_FINAL.pdf

Courts, R., Brophy, L., Bleue, M., Jacques, M., & Badcock, J. C. (2024). Mapping social work's response to the 'grand challenge' of loneliness: A systematic scoping review of the literature. *The British Journal of Social Work, 54*(2), 817–837.

Cuboniks, L. (2018). *The Xenofeminist manifesto: A politics for alienation*. Verso Books. http://www.laboriacuboniks.net/#interrupt

Datar, S., & Bowler, C. N. (2015). Design thinking and innovative problem solving. In J. Canals (Ed.), *Shaping entrepreneurial mindsets: Innovation and entrepreneurship in leadership development* (pp. 119–138). Palgrave Macmillan UK.

Davies, J. (2021). *Sedated: How modern capitalism created our mental health crisis*. Atlantic Books.

Depounti, I., Saukko, P., & Natale, S. (2023). Ideal technologies, ideal women: AI and gender imaginaries in redditors' discussions on the Replika bot girlfriend. *Media, Culture & Society, 45*(4), 720–736.

D'ignazio, C., & Klein, L. F. (2020). *Data feminism*. MIT Press. https://doi.org/10.7551/mitpress/11805.001.0001

Djamasbi, S., Tullis, T., Hsu, J., Mazuera, E., Osberg, K., & Bosch, J. (2007). Gender preferences in web design: Usability testing through eye tracking. *AMCIS 2007 Proceedings* (p. 133). http://aisel.aisnet.org/amcis2007/133

Donovan, D., Furber, G., Cothren, A., Andrew, J., & Gwilt, I. (2022). Visualizing mental health: Co-design for innovative mental health promotion prototypes through interdisciplinary collaboration between psychology professionals, communication design students and tertiary design educators. *Design for Health, 6*(6), 163–184. https://doi.org/10.1080/24735132.2022.2096789

Eltahawy, L., Essig, T., Myszkowski, N., & Trub, L. (2024). Can robots do therapy?: Examining the efficacy of a CBT bot in comparison with other behavioral intervention technologies in alleviating mental health symptoms. *Computers in Human Behavior: Artificial Humans, 2*(1), 100035.

Feminist Internet, & Young, J. (n.d.). https://ugc.futurelearn.com/uploads/files/16/b0/16b088ad-6145-45eb-b5d8-3753a41b4b88/2-10_FeministDesignTool_2.0.pdf

Feminist Principles of the Internet. (n.d.). https://feministinternet.org/index.php/en

Figueroa, C., Luop, T., Aguilera, A., & Lyles, C. (2021). The need for feminist intersectionality in digital health. *The Lancet Digital Health, 3*(8), 526–533. https://doi.org/10.1016/s2589-7500(21)00118-7

Fitzpatrick, K. K., Darcy, A., & Vierhile, M. (2017). Delivering cognitive behavioural therapy to young adults via smartphone: A randomized controlled trial of Woebot. *Cognitive Behaviour Therapy, 46*(4), 201–214.

Foucault, M. (1967). *Madness and civilization: A history of insanity in the age of reason*. Routledge.

Gartner, J. (2024). How much does IT app development cost in Australia? *White Peak Digital*. https://www.whitepeakdigital.com/blog/app-development-cost-australia/

Jarldorn, M., & Emery, S. (2024). Using radical co-design to create and develop a technology-based-solution to improve post-release outcomes for formerly incarcerated women: LindaBot. *International Journal of Communication, 18*, 1246–1265. https://ijoc.org/index.php/ijoc/article/view/21208/4503

Kavanagh, B. E., Corney, K. B., Beks, H., Williams, L., Quirk, S., & Versace, V. (2023). A scoping review of the barriers and facilitators to accessing and utilising mental health services across regional, rural, and remote Australia. *BMC Health Services Research, 23*(1), 1060. https://doi.org/10.1186/s12913-023-10034-4

Kaveladze, B. T., Wasil, A. R., Bunyi, J. B., Ramirez, V., & Schueller, S. M. (2022). User experience, engagement, and popularity in mental health apps: Secondary analysis of app analytics and expert app reviews. *JMIR Human Factors, 9*(1), e30766. https://doi.org/10.2196/30766

Kemp, K. (2024, August 26). Why is it so hard to cancel subscriptions or end 'free' trials? Report shows how companies trap you into paying. *The Conversation*. https://theconversation.com/why-is-it-so-hard-to-cancel-subscriptions-or-end-free-trials-report-shows-how-companies-trap-you-into-paying-237236

Khawaja, Z., & Bèlisle-Pipon, J. (2024, April 28). Your AI therapist is not your therapist: The dangers of relying on AI mental health chatbots. *The Conversation*. https://theconversation.com/your-ai-therapist-is-not-your-therapist-the-dangers-of-relying-on-ai-mental-health-chatbots-225411

Kissling, E. A. (2006). *Capitalizing on the curse: The business of menstruation*. Lynne Rienner Publishers.

Kökçinar, R. (2022). Climate change-related distress within the dominant mental health paradigm: Problems, pitfalls, and a possible way forward. *Psychotherapy and Counselling Journal of Australia, 10*(2). https://doi.org/10.59158/001c.71204

Lau, N., Kola, L., Zhao, X., Asafo, S., Attah, D., & Ben-Zeev, D. (2025). mHealth formental health: Expanding the reach of care. *The Handbook of Mental Health Communication*, 193–205.

Lewis, Z., Pritting, L., Picazo, A., & JeanMarie-Tucker, M. (2020). The utility of wearable fitness trackers and implications for increased engagement: An exploratory, mixed methods observational study. *DIGITAL HEALTH, 6*. https://doi.org/10.1177/2055207619900059

Ludlow, K., Russell, J. K., Ryan, B., Brown, R. L., Joynt, T., Uhlmann, L. R., Smith, G. E., Donovan, C., Hides, L., Spence, S. H., March, S., & Cobham, V. E. (2023). Co-designing a digital mental health platform, "momentum", with young people aged 7–17: A qualitative study. *DIGITAL HEALTH, 9*. https://doi.org/10.1177/20552076231216410

Madianou, M. (2021). Nonhuman humanitarianism: When 'AI for good' can be harmful. *Information, Communication & Society, 24*(6), 850–868.

Mathiason, J. L. (2023). Femtech: The "smart" business of menstruation, hormone tracking, and the corporate construction of risk. *Feminist Studies, 49*(1), 118–149. https://doi.org/10.1353/fem.2023.a901596

McMillan, C. (2022). Monitoring female fertility through 'Femtech': The need for a whole-system approach to regulation. *Medical Law Review, 30*(3), 410–433.

Morgan, A. J., Wright, J., & Reavley, N. J. (2021). Review of Australian initiatives to reduce stigma towards people with complex mental illness: What exists and what works? *International Journal of Mental Health Systems, 15*(1). https://doi.org/10.1186/s13033-020-00423-1

Muchamore, I., Karanikolas, P., & Gooding, P. (2024). How lived experience expertise shapes research and development in digital mental health—A review of literature and insights. *SSRN Electronic Journal*. https://doi.org/10.2139/ssrn.4932039

Mullan, J. (2023). *Decolonizing therapy: Oppression, historical trauma, and politicizing your practice*. WW Norton & Company.
Newcomb, M. (2021). Self-care rhetoric in neoliberal organisations: Social worker experiences. *Practice, 34*(3), 223–238. https://doi.org/10.1080/09503153.2021.1998414
O'Connor, C. A., Zufferey, C., & de Anstiss, H. (2025). Governing failed neoliberal subjects: Representations of women's mental health in Australian mental health policies. *Qualitative Social Work, 24*(1), 61–77. https://doi.org/10.1177/14733250231222020
Orlowski, S., Lawn, S., Venning, A., Winsall, M., Jones, G., Wyld, K., Damarell, R., Antezana, G., Schrader, G., Smith, D., Collin, P., & Bidargaddi, N. (2015). Participatory research as one piece of the puzzle: A systematic review of consumer involvement in design of technology-based youth mental health and well-being interventions. *JMIR Human Factors, 2*(2), e12. https://doi.org/10.2196/humanfactors.4361
Palmer, V., Weavell, W., Callander, R., Piper, D., Richard, L., Maher, L., Boyd, H., Herrman, H., Furler, J., Gunn, J., Iedema, R., & Robert, G. (2019). The participatory zeitgeist: An explanatory theoretical model of change in an era of coproduction and codesign in healthcare improvement. *Medical Humanities, 45*(3), 247–257. https://doi.org/10.1136/medhum-2017-011398
Postmus, J. L., Hoge, G. L., Breckenridge, J., Sharp-Jeffs, N., & Chung, D. (2020). Economic abuse as an invisible form of domestic violence: A multicountry review. *Trauma, Violence, & Abuse, 21*(2), 261–283. https://doi.org/10.1177/1524838018764160
Rapp, A., & Cena, F. (2016). Personal informatics for everyday life: How users without prior self-tracking experience engage with personal data. *International Journal of Human-Computer Studies, 94*, 1–17. https://doi.org/10.1016/j.ijhcs.2016.05.006
Reid, C., Ponic, P., Hara, L., LeDrew, R., Kaweesi, C., & Besla, K. (2011). Living an ethical agreement: Negotiating confidentiality and harm in a feminist participatory action research project. In G. Creese & W. Frisby (Eds.), *Feminist methodologies in community research* (pp. 189–209). University of British Columbia.
Reuters. (2025, May 20). Italy's data watchdog fines AI company Replika's developer $5.6 million. *Reuters*. https://www.reuters.com/sustainability/boards-policy-regulation/italys-data-watchdog-fines-ai-company-replikas-developer-56-million-2025-05-19/
Scholten, H., & Granic, I. (2019). Use of the principles of design thinking to address limitations of digital mental health interventions for youth: Viewpoint. *Journal of Medical Internet Research, 21*(1), 1–14. https://doi.org/10.2196/11528

Snoswell, C., Snoswell, A., & Neil, L. (2025, June 11). Do you talk to AI when you're feeling down? Here's where chatbots get their therapy advice. *The Conversation.* https://theconversation.com/do-you-talk-to-ai-when-youre-feeling-down-heres-where-chatbots-get-their-therapy-advice

Stuart, H. (2021). Professional inefficacy is the exact opposite of the passionate social worker: Discursive analysis of neoliberalism within the writing on self-care in social work. *Journal of Progressive Human Services, 32*(1), 1–16. https://doi.org/10.1080/10428232.2020.1790715

Taylor, J. (2023). *Indicative trauma impact manual.* Victim Focus.

Tsichla, E., Hatzithomas, L., & Boutsouki, C. (2016). Gender differences in the interpretation of web atmospherics: A selectivity hypothesis approach. *Journal of Marketing Communications, 22*(6), 563–586. https://doi.org/10.1080/13527266.2014.903507

van der Westhuizen, D., Conrad, N., Douglas, T., & Mutsvangwa, T. (2020). Engaging communities on health innovation: Experiences in implementing design thinking. *International Quarterly of Community Health Education., 41*(1), 101–114. https://doi.org/10.1177/0272684x19900880

Villatte, A., Pichè, G., Habib, R., & Garièpy, J. (2023). Evaluation of a mental-health literacy and self-care website intended for young people who have a parent with a mental illness. *Advances in Mental Health*, 1–20.

Vu, K., Proctor, R., & Garcia, F. (2021). Website design and evaluation. In G. Salvendy (Ed.), *Handbook of human factors and ergonomics* (4th ed., pp. 1323–1353). John Wiley & Sons.

Website Design Recommended Resources

Beaird, J., Walker, A., & George, J. (2020). *The principles of beautiful web design* (4th ed.). SitePoint Pty Ltd.

Feminist Internet, & Young, J. (n.d.). https://ugc.futurelearn.com/uploads/files/16/b0/16b088ad-6145-45eb-b5d8-3753a41b4b88/2-10_FeministDesignTool_2.0.pdf

Feminist Principles of the Internet. (n.d.). https://feministinternet.org/index.php/en

Krug, S. (2006). *Don't make me think!: A common sense approach to web usability* (2nd ed.).

CHAPTER 7

Embedding Collaborators' Voices into Co-Design: Reflecting on the Project

Kizzy Yang, Rosie Dale, Abbey Hood, Jasmine Lloyd, Kate Deuter, Michele Jarldorn, and Nicole Moulding

Abstract This final chapter brings together our insights from conducting the project. Four of the young women who participated in across every stage of the project join us as co-authors as they document their journeys of participation. The chapter is metaphorically framed by a series of 'destination points', represented by five different platforms in a train station. The young women were supported to recall their experiences using a

K. Yang
Freshwater, NSW, Australia

R. Dale
Glenelg, SA, Australia

A. Hood
Mount Barker, SA, Australia

J. Lloyd
Chelsea, VIC, Australia

K. Deuter · M. Jarldorn · N. Moulding
University of South Australia, Magill, SA, Australia
e-mail: Kate.Deuter@unisa.edu.au;
Michele.jarldorn@unisa.edu.au; Nicole.Moulding@unisa.edu.au

M. Jarldorn et al. (eds.), *Feminist Action Research in Mental Health*, https://doi.org/10.1007/978-3-032-04406-8_7

research journey template designed by a research team member. Framed around the concept of a train journey, each platform transports the young women back through the project, stopping at each of the co-design destinations they visited along the way. Here, the aim was to prompt deep reflection about their experiences throughout the life of the project: Platform 1—an online survey exploring young women's experience of mental health peer support; Platform 2—online focus groups exploring the meaning of peer support; Platform 3—co-design workshops to develop the website wireframe; Platform 4—finalising the website, and Platform 5—launching the website. We enhance the chapter with a discussion around the politics of co-authorship and the benefits of participating in feminist research.

Keywords Research participant co-authorship • Inclusive participation • Co-production of knowledge

Introduction

The relational aspect of co-design requires a respectful closure that recognises participants' contributions much further than the exchange of honorariums or shopping vouchers. As Hutchinson (2024) explains "relationships are central to knowledge production and [that] people with lived experience are valid knowers" (p. 5). Co-design, and participatory action-oriented research require *meaningful* inclusion rather than representation throughout the entire process. Meaningful involvement in participatory research requires taking the time to build rapport and relationships and takes "effort on the part of both the researcher and the participant" (Pope, 2020, p. 3749). Yet, typically, as a project comes to an end, the grant report and budget acquittal are submitted, and the researchers then publish what they learned. Although idealistically, publishing from research is beneficial to society as it extends knowledge, as Jarldorn and Gatwiri (2022) explain "without publications, acquiring a space in academia would be impossible" (p. 535), thus ensuring that often, the greatest benefit is afforded to researchers, rather than participants. A quick online search of the question 'what are the benefits of publishing from academic research?' provided the following answer: building a career, proving that your research has merit and contributing to scholarly debate. Then surely it would follow that if participants were truly being valued for their contributions, then they would be invited to contribute to publishing endeavours.

One of the aspects of participatory and co-design research that receives minimal attention is how participants' voices can truly be acknowledged and honoured through publication and authorship (Jarldorn, 2022). Writing about doing action research, Cherry (2010) argues that researchers require a commitment to "stay in the action and not retreat to the margins where they write intense, anguished reflective pieces about their difficulties but accomplish little" (p. 239). Yet, 15 years later, Phillips et al. (2022) propose that examples of "co-authorship by co-researchers and academic researchers are rare...despite the documented benefits to co-researchers and their communities" (p. 2).

When consulting our university's policies on responsible practice in research (UniSA, 2024), the criterion for authorship is that there should be a scholarly contribution to a minimum of one, but preferably two or more of the following dot points. We have presented the aspects of these that we believe our participants met in bold:

- conception and **design of the** project or **output**
- acquisition of research data where the acquisition has required significant intellectual judgement, planning, **design, or input**
- **contribution of knowledge**, where justified, including Indigenous knowledge
- analysis or **interpretation of research data**
- **drafting significant parts of the research output or critically revising it so as to contribute to its interpretation.**

For researchers seeking to explore and build the knowledge base of the discrete aspects of co-design, a policy analysis of how authorship policies can be applied to participants could be useful in advancing co-design practices. This idea is supported by the journal editors of *Affilia*, whose recent editorial on positionality (Jackson et al., 2024) included a list of 15 points for consideration (see Chap. 4 for a more detailed discussion). Specific to authorship, they ask; "Is the first author from the community of focus?" and "If the current manuscript emerged from participatory action research, community-based participatory research, or another engaged research effort, have community collaborators been included in authorship?" (pp. 8–9). However, as academics for whom writing is part and parcel of our terms of employment, it is important to consider how we support participants to co-author that does not make the task overwhelming or a chore.

Creative Methods to Support Co-Authorship

When the research team met to reflect upon what we learned from the project and discuss the development of this book, we contemplated how we could support the young women who worked with us to co-design the website across the project to co-author the final chapter in this book. They had indicated they were excited to contribute to a chapter but weren't sure where to begin. Our project research associate, Kate, developed a research journey template that was representative of our two-year journey of learning and collaboration. Across the following pages, you'll see how the women used the template to reflect upon their experience of contributing to the project. We have interspersed the young women's responses to the template prompts throughout the final section of this chapter.

However, before we do, it is worth pausing to consider how co-authorship has been achieved in other research projects. We were surprised at the dearth of publications on the politics of co-authorship with research participants, with most tangentially addressing co-authorship without describing *how* it was achieved. One of the better examples we found reports on a project that explored the benefits of dance for couples where one member of the couple has been diagnosed with Parkinson's disease (Phillips et al., 2022). To co-author their paper, the academic research team used 'collaborative autoethnography' as a method, creating a 'suggested roadmap' to ensure that their co-authors understood the process of developing the publication. While there are some similarities in language between their idea of a roadmap and Kate's idea of a train journey, the authors recorded an interview with co-design participants to ask specific questions and then used letter writing between the research team and the participants to ground their argument. Later, excerpts of the recorded interviews and full, verbatim texts of the exchanged letters were entered into the publication.

At the forefront of Kate's idea for developing the 'train journey' template was the notion of 'stepping back in time', which was critical given the iterative approach to data collection and analysis and the actual length of engagement in the study. In this way, we invited the young women to 'go back' and reflect on their experience of each stage of the project, this is how idea of taking a train journey—'back in time'—was realised. Kate located a series of five images on iStock™, each depicting a young woman waiting on a train station platform. From there, each image was assigned to a 'platform' leading to a 'destination' (i.e., online survey, online focus group, co-design workshop, and so on). Across the following pages, we present excerpts from the reflections provided by our co-authors, Kizzy, Rosie, Abbey and Jasmine.

Each young woman was provided with a draft copy of this chapter and invited to provide feedback, which has been incorporated into the final work.

What Did the Young Women Say?

The first section of the research journey template began by providing an overview of the project. We reminded participants about the theoretical framework used in the project and the specific aims of the survey. Each were invited to request a copy of their survey responses.

Okay! Here we go ...

PLATFORM 1

Destination: SURVEY

We're about get on board. You'll need to cast your mind RIGHT BACK now! You might remember the survey that included quantitative questions (in these, we asked you to give a rating) and qualitative questions (where we invited you to provide richer, personal descriptions of your experiences). This survey was open nationally to people who identify as women or non-binary aged 18–30 years old. You completed this survey online sometime between June and September 2021 (yes, it was that long ago now!), along with fifty-one other young women.

Co-Author Reflections

Kizzy: I remember feeling very empowered by the research study and questions—I felt like I was a part of something with a lot of potential, something that could become big and really meaningful, and that felt very exciting. It's not very often I'm asked about my experiences with mental health support specifically as a young female—I often feel my struggles have gone unnoticed or unidentified. I felt like I was exactly who they wanted information from and that felt both weird and special—I was their target population—they wanted information from young women like me with mental health challenges—it felt like such a novel experience.

Looking back on my survey responses I am surprised by how much specific and varied information I gave—I identified many things that I found helpful that surprised me. I think the way the questions were worded really allowed me to explore aspects of my mental health and healing (and the barriers) in a way that I often don't get the opportunity to explore.

I felt empowered by all the questions that were specific to young women and that were gender specific—it felt like I was finally being seen and someone was actually interested in me and my experiences as a young woman with mental health challenges. Weirdly, it had never occurred to me that there wasn't really much out there for young women's mental health in Australia and online, and just not much gender-specific information. It was something I'd never even considered to be possible or that I could ask for. This survey helped me realise how significant of a gap this was and how many of us had been suffering in silence and masking to get by, just as I had throughout most of my school years and most of my years in uni and early work. In my last years of high school I was having panic attacks, hallucinating, and having delusions, all of which went unnoticed. I wasn't once referred to the school counsellor due to mental health concerns and had no clue how much I was suffering. I was constantly blaming and criticising myself. I hated myself for how I was feeling and had no clue that it was in fact the systems around me that had very much failed me and left me to suffer on my own—especially since I was underage when I went through one of my greatest periods of suffering. The second time around I was an early-career speech therapist and had the privilege of being empowered by some knowing of the health system and could get myself into a mental health service, that later became the gateway to discovering the depths of my challenges and the breadth of supports I could access. However, none of the services were specifically for young women.

My final survey response surprised me—I actually mentioned that whilst I thought it was important for young women to be involved in the design of the online support, that men should still be involved for diversity. I strongly disagree with that now. They have no place and no say in this matter. In fact it's difficult to accept I even wrote that back then. I wonder if this was due to my own internalised sexism and also feelings of inferiority or fear of perhaps asking for "too much" as a young woman—feeling like it wasn't possible to ask for something to be purely made for young women and by women. I'm reminded of a time when I told a female friend of mine that I was attending a women-only community centre, men weren't allowed to attend—she responded with a look of disgust and shared her opinion of how ridiculous and unnecessary it was. I felt so much shame wash over me at that response. I now feel really quite angry about it too. My horrible experiences with men give me every right to proudly attend a place that is just for women. However, her response made me much more careful—I stopped sharing about me attending this place as openly as before.

Jasmine: I never would have thought that doing a lived experience of mental health survey, through COVID lockdown times for me in Melbourne, would have led to so many extra opportunities. I'm very grateful to have found this study and the lovely women in research running it. As well as us group of women consumers that have something to say about women's mental health from our own everyday life.

Abbey: My adolescence had been plagued by mental health challenges and I had made several attempts over the past decade to engage with mental health services although I never found one that felt genuine, or safe. I had gone through the process again in 2020, (the GP, the MHCP, the medication) and the same patterns emerged. The feeling of not being understood by practitioners is unfortunately too common in mental health services. As a woman, being perceived as capable often feels essential, not only for personal validation but also to protect against judgements that might lead to intrusive scrutiny or assumptions about my ability to care for myself and my family. And as a single parent there's often additional vulnerability in how problems can be perceived and, at times, weaponised against you. Issues such as stress, financial challenges, or mental health struggles are too easily misinterpreted as inadequacies or risks, rather than seen as natural responses to complex circumstances.

To this day, I am still reluctant to engage with mental health services due to the impact this could have on my career, and on my family. When the opportunity arose to share my experiences anonymously, I took it. I never expected it to lead to anything more, I just thought maybe sharing my experience would help somebody somewhere think a little deeper about why our mental health system sucks and often fails the people that need it most.

Okay. Whenever you're ready, let's head to our next destination ...

PLATFORM 2

Destination: ONLINE FOCUS GROUPS

Everyone who completed the survey was invited to provide a contact phone number and/or email address if they were interested in participating further in an online focus group.

Did you know? Twenty-one young women volunteered to be involved in this next stage.

You were one of them.

After you were all contacted, you and ten other young women agreed and participated in an online focus group. We analysed the survey dataset and drilled down to some specific areas that we wanted to explore further with you and other young women in those online focus groups.

Co-Author Reflections

Abbey: I was surprised and curious when I was contacted to participate in this study further. Feminism is a concept I am aware of and identify with, but I had not ever engaged with a group of individuals with a shared goal so engrained in the theory. Empowerment and mutuality became a prominent theme in the project from day one.

Payment for our time and contributions was also an important factor in my agreement to proceed. Lived experience is often sought after and treated as a valuable asset to enhance the delivery of mental health services, but it's frequently undervalued when it comes to actual compensation. While organisations regularly promote lived experience as a unique selling point, they rarely compensate it at the level of formal qualifications or academic experience.

Kizzy: Everyone got to have their say and it didn't feel clinical—we all seemed to be respected as individuals with expertise. I felt empowered by how anything I said, and any of the other young women said, was respected and heard—this felt so weird and precious as I, possibly also due to my cultural background, had often felt invisible and my opinions ignored due to my age, gender, race and appearance—it was weird to have every little thing no matter how small taken seriously. I enjoyed the intimacy of the small group and the quietly burning passion in some of the attendees.

It was so inspiring to see the facilitators/researchers talk about feminism with such passion and without fear of consequence or shame—something I so rarely see. It felt like a very safe space—I sometimes like to think about the women's communities of our ancestors who would gather in circles, just women, share wisdom and heal together. When I think of peer support, I think of safety and belonging—the feeling that I'm not alone and that I have empowered women who have my back—that we share a common goal and experience.

Women mask so well, we know how to blend in and use a high level of compensatory strategies to seem "normal" or "okay"—we're expected from a young age to seem in control and gentle or quiet—we're trained to behave in acceptable ways—I think this, along with perhaps research that (I think) is mainly done on white men, mean it is so much more difficult to spot when young women are suffering and need support—perhaps there's also that element of sexism where women's problems are dismissed more—I certainly never ever felt safe enough to talk about my mental health with anyone as a young female—I just didn't think anyone would believe me or take me seriously or that they would perhaps take me too seriously and that would lead to problems like being sent to a mental health ward.

Peer support for me would also be around redefining what is normal, or different but not bad or shameful—and knowing that there is help—help for when you don't want to engage in the formal supports that could perhaps have more serious consequences too.

Rosie: I've found that many projects that ask for lived experience input still tend to be one-of opportunities. They've often been more about consulting than co-design, where people with lived experience provide input based on something pre-existing, rather than being able to plan and build something from the ground up—all the way from the beginning to the end. In my opinion, the latter yields better results, but it's also much more empowering and interesting for the participant—I speak from first-hand experience!

We got to talk about and explore in online focus groups what we found were important issues facing us as young women, and the benefits of peer support. We acknowledged the impact of gender-based aspects on women's mental health and wellbeing, such as domestic violence, body image issues, misogyny, systemic dismissal of physical health problems, and societal pressure.

It's always nice when what you share is echoed by others. I found it fulfilling to be in a space with mutual understanding while also getting to hear inspiring ideas and insightful viewpoints. In these focus groups I got to discuss the universality of lived experiences, even if on a surface level they don't appear the same. I always try to remember that my painful, embarrassing, and shameful emotions and thoughts were experienced by many others. Mutually sharing stories of struggling and healing can help people to bond.

And another thing: At times, it can be awkward to talk about pay, but I think remuneration is an important part of a collaborative process and of any process where people with lived experience are consulted. Whether it be prepaid debit cards or a casual hourly rate, getting financially reimbursed for time spent and expertise shared is another way that participants such as myself can feel genuinely valued. It indicates to us that our involvement is taken seriously, and it also creates a sense of personal ownership in the project.

Okay, we're heading off again now to our next destination ...

PLATFORM 3

Destination: ONLINE CO-DESIGN WORKSHOPS

*In this section of the research journey template, screenshots of the online co-design workshop exercises where we used Miro were included in the document.

What we did:

The combined findings from the survey and online focus groups led the conduct of two online **co-design** workshops with you and the other young women who participated in the focus groups. The online co-design workshops were co-facilitated by Nicole, Michele, and Kate and Jane Andrew. You might remember Jane was also joined by a Match Studio former Masters' student Pooja Kagrana, who brought high-level website design skills to the project.

Together, we created a wireframe (or a basic shell) of a website, incorporating your suggestions along with some of the ideas proposed in the earlier survey and focus groups. The wireframe was informed by design principles to align with what the finished website might look like, but without the full functionality that requires the specialist skills of a qualified computer programmer. To create the website prototype, we used Wix™ software that provides cloud-based web development services. It allows users to create HTML5 websites and mobile sites through the use of online drag and drop tools. During the co-design workshops, the design tool Miro™ was used to provide a collaborative, online platform for you to contribute to the creation of a virtual whiteboard. In preparation for the first workshop, you were encouraged to visit the Miro™ site to familiarise yourself with our private workshop white board space. In addition to the combined survey and focus group findings, the direction of the online co-design workshops was guided by the following three mental health design-related questions:

(i) How can an online support platform increase mental health awareness and destigmatise mental health difficulties?
(ii) How can an online support platform cope with feelings of insecurity, doubt and judgement?
(iii) How can an online support platform make professional help for mental health approachable?

In the first exercise, you were orientated to a range of potential features of an online mHealth site. Remember doing this exercise?! In adopting the 'Rose/Thorn/Bud' template, you were invited to think about and assign features to each area. You were also invited to think beyond the present list of features to include any other features you had seen elsewhere, particularly those pertinent to younger women's needs and/or peer support.

In the second workshop, you were invited to further prioritise (from 1 to 5) those features that were prioritised in the first workshop as critical components for the new website wireframe prototype. Next, you were invited to 'consider all things representative of the look and feel of a [successful] online mental health portal. Based on pre-selection of four existing online mental health sites, including an internationally based mindfulness/meditation site and a major national Australian mental health site, Jane and Pooja engaged you and the other young women in conversation about the elements of the four sites that you liked and/or disliked.

These were the most frequently discussed ideas:

1. Security—Quick Exit, Face ID. Silent notification—silence response.
2. Language and education—inclusive and accessible medical knowledge.
3. The ability to talk to experienced people.
4. Related community intended discussions, individualised discussion groups.
5. Chat bot—available at suitable reach
6. Interactive—wellbeing activities where people can share their experiences, e.g., upload photos/artworks and see others' uploads too.
7. Accessible—access to text being read out loud in lots of languages, available in simple English.
8. Images of humans are not Photoshopped.
9. Help in navigating the mental health system and also support/guidance to trauma informed legal advice if pressing charges.
10. Easy to navigate, not too much text. Videos, images audio, podcasts, short stories.

Developing a Personalised Mood Board

During the final activity, the young women were presented with a wide variety of images and of varying colours, shapes and themes and some text-based phrases and invited to make selections to create their own, personalised 'mood board'. The aim of the final two exercises was to identify any commonalities associated among the young women's preferences for the general aesthetic of the website.

Here is yours ...

Your Mood Board:

*Each of the young women were provided with a copy of their personalised mood board to assist them in reflecting on this stage of the project.

Collaborative reflection

At the end of the second workshop, you were informed about and invited to take part [subject to funding outcomes] in the next proposed stage of the study where we planned to take the wireframe prototype to full functionality and identify hosts and/or sponsors. All of you expressed an interest in participating in this next stage. In late 2022, additional funding was secured to commence the project at the start of 2023. YAAAAYYY!!! Five of you who participated in the first stage collaborated with us on this next stage.

Co-Author Reflections

Kizzy: Being part of the process of coming up with resources and content for the website was fun and also somewhat overwhelming—it felt like we were starting from scratch and that there was so much potential and yet at the same time not a lot out there that would be easily accessible for the website. I felt my perfectionism and fear of saying the wrong thing come up quite a few times and had to remind myself that anything and everything was okay—that I was just sharing my thoughts and ideas—this was a safe space.

It was so wonderful to see things to completion—I was impressed at how quickly the project ended—it felt like it could go on and on—the website was far from perfect but was looking very promising—others showed interest in it and wanted to take it on—I saw proof of how things don't need to be perfect, they can be imperfect and incomplete yet still appreciated and supported by other women.

Later, when we had co-design workshops, we got to collaborate on what we would find helpful or unhelpful on the online support platform, drawing from our own experiences of what elements we found significant, both now and in the past. Online mental health resources are often just a list of helplines, so we wanted something that was easy to use, accessible, and engaging. Since it was co-design, we could aim as high as we wanted.

Abbey: I found it difficult to envision what the website was going to be. Everybody had fantastic ideas. During the development phase I felt overwhelmed by the scope of possibilities. I felt strongly that we needed to ensure a uniqueness to our project as the world of online mental health support is already vast and repetitive. We were provided the opportunity to make ongoing contributions, including of our own imagery. The website was very much designed to communicate hope, support, and safety, and to feel relatable, helping users feel understood and seen. I think we all knew creating something distinctive would be challenging, but it was essential to ensure the website was simple, welcoming, user-friendly, and, above all, safe.

I felt strongly that the website needed to be a platform rich in resources and information, offering more than just symbolic messaging. Over the course of the project, we refined our ideas, discussed the limitations and functionality of what we could deliver and established peer2me.

Okay, we have nearly arrived at our final destination ...!

PLATFORM 4

Destination: FINALISING THE WEBSITE

Following the workshops, we met with the young women and took them through the wireframe prototype informed by their ideas and preferences as expressed in the focus groups and survey. From their feedback, we learned that they wanted even more diversity in the images used, ones that were not airbrushed as is typical of images available for use within website development programs such as Wix™, the program used to create the wireframe.

Co-Author Reflection

Rosie: When talking about the design and appearance of the platform, us participants got a bit vocal about the stock images of women that were suggested! There's still too much airbrushing and Photoshop[ing] out there. It makes a difference to see an image of a woman who actually looks like you would on an average day.

PLATFORM 4, continued ...

In our final co-design sessions, we worked with web developer Kirstie Wyatt, to finalise our website prototype. Kirstie has heaps of experience in website design, she does this for her own business but also teaches website design at university. First up, she shifted our website wireframe onto WordPress. Kirstie said this was because of its superior functionality. We also created a team **Trello**, which we used as a shared repository for ideas and resources for the website. As a group, we met with Kirstie a few times to see how the website was progressing and to provide feedback. We spent a lot of time deliberating over the name of the site, and choosing how it would look. As Kirstie shared her screen with us in these meetings, we could see what goes on behind the scenes of building a website.

Co-Author Reflections

Kizzy: Regarding the search terms I'd use, if I'm being completely honest, I've never really used gendered terms when looking for information on mental health and trauma—I don't expect to find it so I've never tried looking for it. I've had to try my best to imagine what it would be like to go looking for mental health information and support specifically for women. For example, some phrases might be: What mental health services are available for women? How do female hormones affect mental health? Mental health supports for women. How to improve my mental wellbeing

Some future articles that would be great to see would include menstrual health, emotional labour in the household, ageing, adulting, body image, and being assertive/knowing what is okay and what is not i.e. disrespectful. And also, how to have a healthy relationship with exercise because quite often the exercise/health movement is presented with weight loss in mind, not health or balance. It would be good if a trans woman could share her journey.

We are now approaching our final destination ...!

PLATFORM 5

Destination: LAUNCHING THE WEBSITE

peer2me

In late November 2023, the website was completed, and we held a hybrid (in person and online) launch and a knowledge exchange for the project. We invited representatives from key organisations and individuals who provide mental health support. We also had a representative from the project funder, The Breakthrough Mental Health Research Foundation attend. Some of you attended in person, and some of you attended online. At the launch, we revisited the steps we took to design and complete the project. The people who came loved hearing about your participation and gave us heaps of positive feedback. We are still in discussions with potential organisations to take carriage of the site.

Co-Author Reflections

Kizzy: I wished I could've been there in person—I wanted to experience the energy of young women being celebrated despite their mental health challenges; however I was so glad I got to be there online and that I was given the opportunity to speak my truth—it was so wonderful to hear my fellow participants speak as well in different forms and in such supported ways.

Before speaking I reached out to one of the researchers as I was feeling anxious about the launch and yet wanted to attend and say something—it was so relieving and encouraging to be told that anything was okay and that I would be supported—they weren't just words either. I experienced it in action, felt the care—before, during, and after the launch.

I didn't once feel like my participation was tokenistic—I had a clear purpose and my thoughts and opinions mattered—the researchers embodied what they were researching—support for young women's mental health.

I didn't think research could be done like this—there was so much action, outcome and tangibility—we've been given so many opportunities to participate, make a difference and be part of something bigger—I think this has definitely raised the bar for me in terms of what research should be like and what we deserve as young women.

Rosie: It does spark joy to reflect on my participation in this project, which lasted over two years, even though it means I can't specifically remember all of the things I said and did! It's been something special to keep seeing the same people over a long period of time in online meetings, and to build connection while coming up with the framework and design for the peer support website. I was fortunate enough to attend the website launch in person in Adelaide. Not only was there free food, but it felt special to see the project come to fruition, and to witness that our feedback had been taken on board and heard. It was a day I could feel proud of my efforts as part of a collective.

Things are slowly easing down now, so I will miss this experience but always be grateful for what it had to offer. We were only a small cohort putting together the platform, so I hope in the future more women will contribute to the website and provide their own unique and diverse insights. I want *peer2me* to continue to become more relevant and helpful for all Australian young women, regardless of their sexuality, gender assigned at birth, cultural identity, background, or faith.

Jasmine: To be able to assist in the initial study, co-design the website, see it go live and now reflect in this book chapter, has been great. Overall, hearing other female's wants in a mental health website for them, and to be able to all collaborate our ideas to become a real working site has been so rewarding. Not to mention the actual positive affects it's had on how I view my own mental health, and feeling so much acceptance and validation of what struggles mentally anyone goes through every day. I think it's a great personal accomplishment for me, and as a response to this gap in peer-to-peer material for women's mental health with a thoroughly researched resource.

I never would have thought that doing a lived experience of mental health survey, through COVID lockdown times for me in Melbourne, would have led to so many extra opportunities.

Abbey: My participation in the project has inspired significant personal and professional growth. Balancing my drive to stay meaningfully engaged in this project with my other commitments was difficult. Imposter syndrome, and the need to feel my contributions were worthwhile became a personal challenge and held me back, particularly during the last stage of the project. When reflecting on my involvement in the development of peer2me and the subsequent publication, I've realised that much of my burnout stems from the high standards I expect myself to meet in each role I take on. These expectations, while motivating, can sometimes be unhealthily high, making it difficult to feel confident and satisfied with my work. The sense of ownership in this project became incredibly motivating in the end, especially in a project where our insights and experiences genuinely shaped the outcome.

Ownership allows you to feel personally invested in the project's success, making it so much more meaningful and rewarding. It became not just about completing a task, a focus group, or a survey—it became about contributing to something that reflects our voices and our values. It's been an excellent learning experience and something I feel proud to share with others. I'm grateful that this group of women saw the worth in what we each had to offer. That collective recognition of each other's value speaks to the power of shared purpose and collaborative work, especially within a group that valued and compensated our lived experience as an essential form of expertise.

Concluding Remarks from the Research Team

As we finalised this last chapter of the book, we were heartened by the young women's willingness to share their observations of participation and contribution. Their testimonies throughout this chapter speak to the importance of offering meaningful involvement in co-design projects and participants being adequately compensated for their contributions. They also reflected positively on the feminist ethics of care used throughout and how they appreciated the development of relationships and sharing of experiences. Overall, their reflections ring true with the observation made by Phillips et al. (2022), in that participatory research practices are "relational practices of mutual learning" (p. 2). Our co-author's responses to the prompts within our research journey template confirmed for us why *doing* co-design grounded in feminist principles has benefits beyond gaining research data, while an unexpected outcome from co-authoring this chapter with us is that two of the co-authors have recently co-authored a book chapter with another of our colleagues about the lived experiences of mental health challenges.

Our co-authors' contributions to this chapter echo the experience of Buchanan and Wendt (2018), who found that women often participate in feminist research as a way to make things better for other women, but in the process of participating, realise that the experience enabled them to reframe their experiences of violence and abuse as stories of survival. Some of the young women's reflections reminded us of the feminist consciousness-raising practices commonly used throughout the second wave of feminism. One of the most useful explanations of the meaning of feminist consciousness-raising can be found within the editor's note embedded in a seminal paper by Catharine MacKinnon (1982), who wrote:

> Central to feminist theory and feminist method Catharine A. MacKinnon shows, is consciousness raising. Through this process, feminists confront the reality of women's condition by examining their experience and by taking this analysis as the starting point for individual and social change. By its nature, this method of inquiry challenges traditional notions of authority and objectivity and opens a dialectical questioning of existing power structures, own experience, and of theory itself. (p. 515)

Since the excitement of the knowledge exchange and website launch, we have met with a few organisations to discuss the potential of them taking carriage of the website as an adjunct to the work they already do. As yet, we have not found a suitable organisation that has the right combination of a commitment to feminist values and staffing resources to maintain the chat and check-in functions the young women wanted. Therefore, the research team are continuing to maintain and update the peer2me website as a useful repository of feminist-informed mental health and wellbeing resources, and as an example of what can be created when researchers and people with living experience work together.

Since we conceptualised the project in late 2020, and began reviewing the literature early in 2021, we have observed an increase in the number of studies and publications on peer-to-peer support around mental health. We also believe that the benefits of co-creating a service, an intervention or a set of resources are not just for the imagined end-users, but that involvement in the co-design process, and being actively involved in creating solutions can in themselves promote mental wellbeing. To access the project website, search 'peer2me', and please use the link on the website to let us know if you have any resources you'd like to share on the site.

References

Buchanan, F., & Wendt, S. (2018). Opening doors: Women's participation in feminist studies about domestic violence. *Qualitative Social Work, 17*(6), 762–777. https://doi.org/10.1177/14733250176940

Cherry, N. (2010). Action research. In J. Higgs, N. Cherry, R. Macklin, & R. Ajjawi (Eds.), *Researching practice: A discourse on qualitative methodologies* (pp. 237–246). Sense Publishers. https://doi.org/10.1163/9789460911835_026

Hutchinson, J. (2024). The gendered, misogynoiristic, and colonial genocidal logics of strip searching. *Affilia, Feminist Inquiry in Social Work*. Online First. https://journals.sagepub.com/doi/full/10.1177/08861099241297153

Jackson, K. F., Goodkind, S., Diaz, M., Karandikar, S., Beltrán, R., Kim, M. E., Zelnick, J. R., Gibson, M. F., Mountz, S., Miranda Samuels, G. E., & Harrell, S. (2024). Positionality in critical feminist scholarship: Situating social locations and power within knowledge production. *Affilia—Feminist Inquiry in Social Work, 39*(1), 5–11. https://doi.org/10.1177/08861099231219848

Jarldorn, M. (2022). Centring participants' voices as inclusive research practice: Putting the voice into photovoice. In P. Liamputtong (Ed.), *Handbook of social inclusion: Research and practices in health and social sciences* (pp. 1–17). Springer International Publishing. https://doi.org/10.1007/978-3-030-89594-5_72

Jarldorn, M., & Gatwiri, K. (2022). Shaking off the imposter syndrome: Our place in the resistance. In *The Palgrave handbook of imposter syndrome in higher education* (pp. 529–543). Springer International Publishing. https://doi.org/10.1007/978-3-030-86570-2_32

MacKinnon, C. A. (1982). Feminism, Marxism, method, and the state: An agenda for theory. *Signs: Journal of Women in Culture and Society, 7*(3), 515–544. https://doi.org/10.1086/493898

Phillips, L., Larsen, A., & Mengel, L. (2022). What "coproduction" in participatory research means from participants' perspectives: A collaborative autoethnographic inquiry. *Journal of Participatory Research Methods, 3*(2). https://doi.org/10.35844/001c.37638

Pope, E. M. (2020). From participants to co-researchers: Methodological alterations to a qualitative case study. *The Qualitative Report, 25*(10), 3749–3761. https://doi.org/10.46743/2160-3715/2020.4394

UniSA. (2024). https://i.unisa.edu.au/policies-and-procedures/university-policies/research/res-12/

Index

M. Jarldorn et al. (eds.), *Feminist Action Research in Mental Health*, https://doi.org/10.1007/978-3-032-04406-8

FSC
www.fsc.org
MIX
Papier | Fördert gute Waldnutzung
FSC® C083411

Kolibri 360 GmbH
Ferdinand-Jühlke-Straße 7
99095 Erfurt, Deutschland
produktsicherheit@kolibri360.de